Hair Style

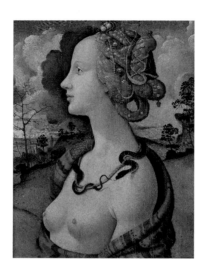

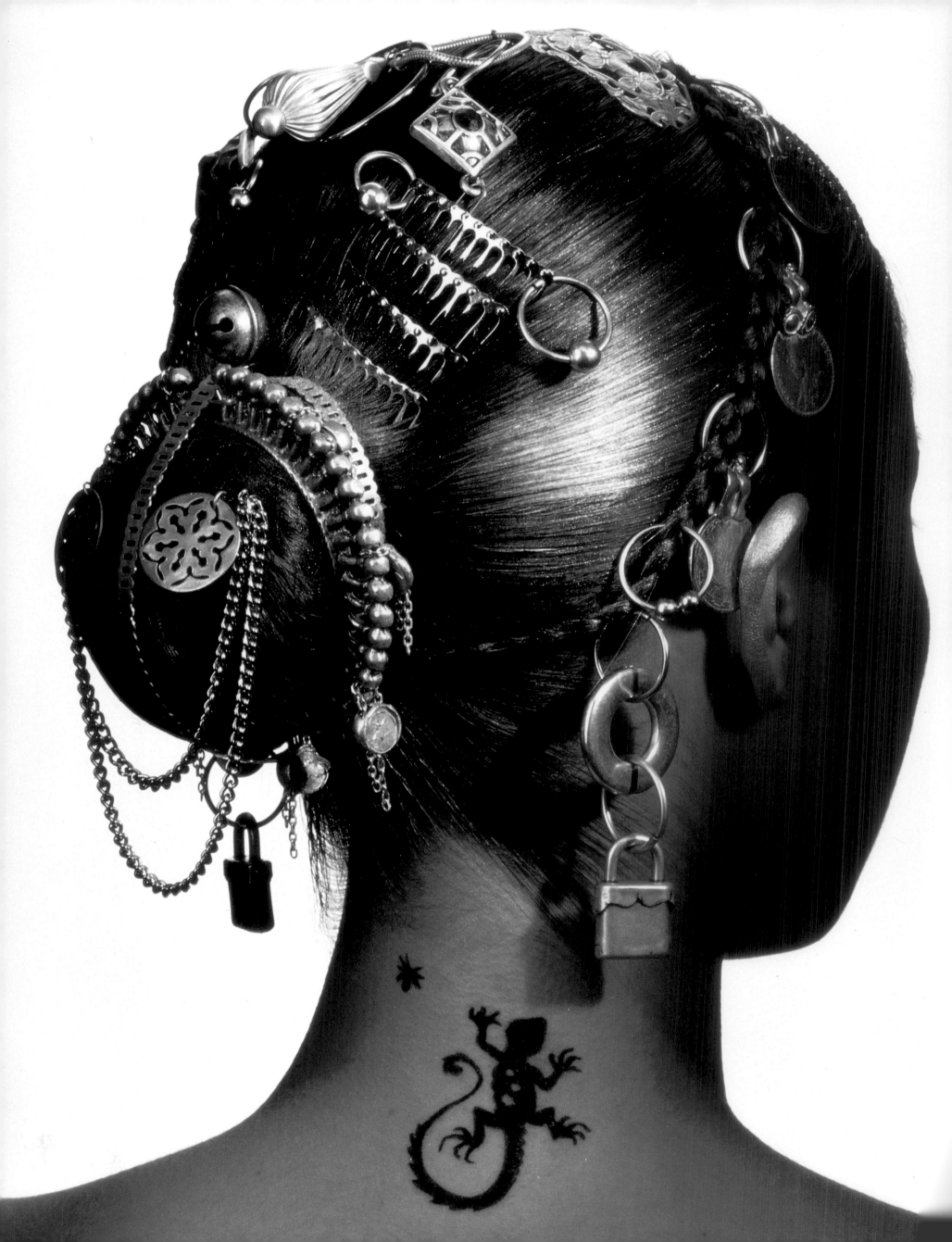

Hair Style
by Amy Fine Collins

Preface by Liz Tilberis

Edited by Antoinette White

Designed by Toshiya Masuda

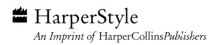 HarperStyle
An Imprint of HarperCollins*Publishers*

HarperCollins*Publishers*/Callaway Editions 1995

To Grandma with the bewitching black bun and Flora with the silky, coppery wisps.

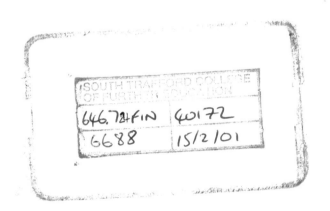
Hair Style copyright ©1995 by Callaway Editions, Inc.

Preface copyright ©1995 by Liz Tilberis

All rights reserved.

The photographs herein which are attributed to named photographers,
except as otherwise noted herein, are copyrighted by the photographers.

No part of this book may be used or reproduced in any manner whatsoever without
written permission of Callaway Editions except in the case of brief quotations embedded
in critical articles and reviews. For information, write HarperCollins*Publishers*, Inc.,
10 East 53rd Street, New York, NY 10022.
HarperCollins books may be purchased for educational, business, or sales promotional use.
For information, write Special Markets Department, HarperCollins*Publishers*, Inc.,
10 East 53rd Street, New York, NY 10022.

First Edition

ISBN 0-06-270145-2

Library of Congress Catalog Card Number 95-37127

95 96 97 98 99 10 9 8 7 6 5 4 3 2 1

Printed in Hong Kong

Half-title page: *La Bella Simonetta* by Piero di Cosimo, c. 1480. Collection Musée Condé, Chantilly, France. Photo RMN

Frontispiece: Susan Gin, with hair styled by Orlando Pita, photographed by Irving Penn for American *Vogue*.
Copyright ©1994 by The Condé Nast Publications Inc.

Linda Evangelista, with hair styled by Didier Malige, photographed by Bruce Weber for Italian *Vogue*. Courtesy Italian *Vogue*

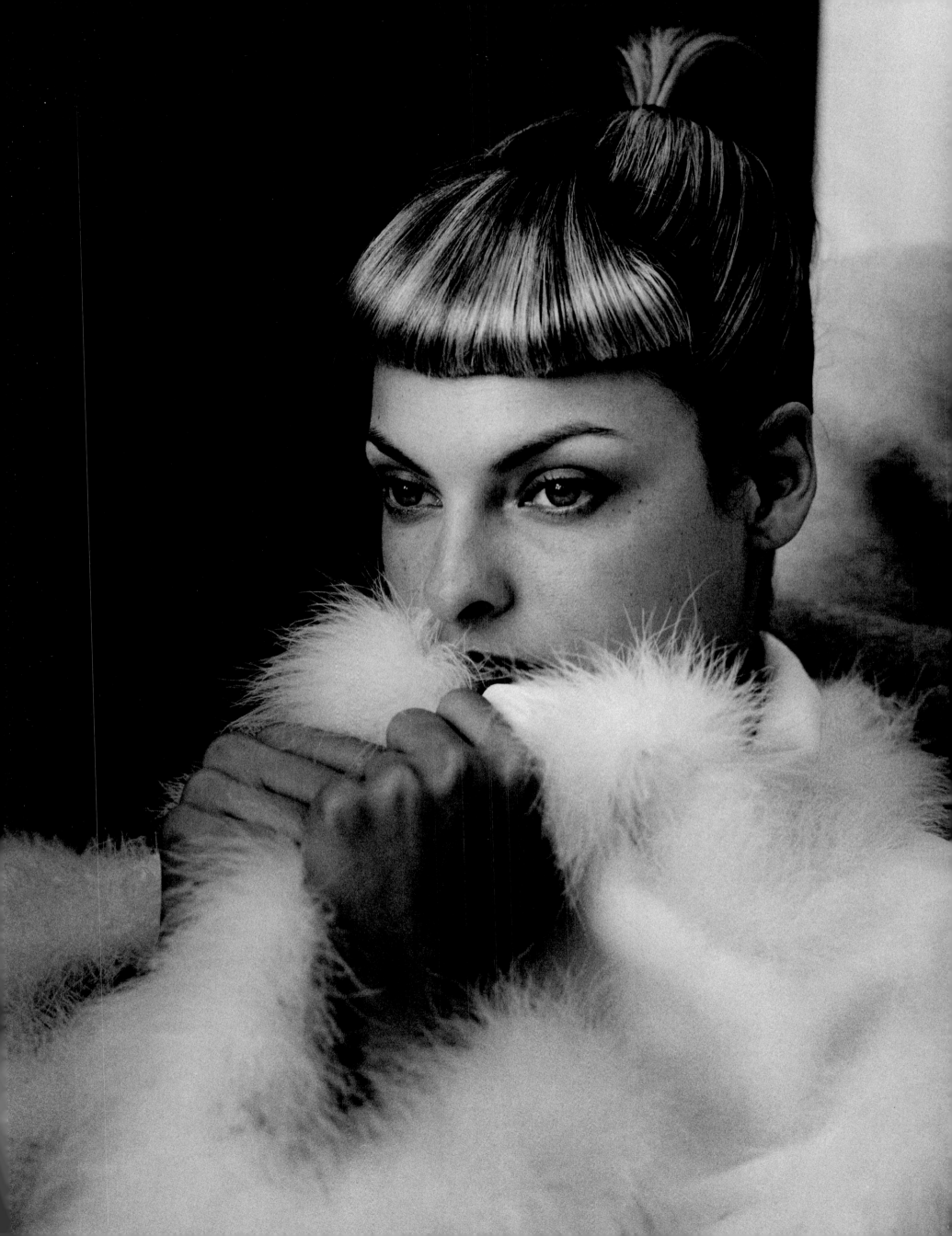

Contents

Janet Jackson, with hair styled by Janet Zeitoun, photographed by Eddie Wolfl for *Vibe*

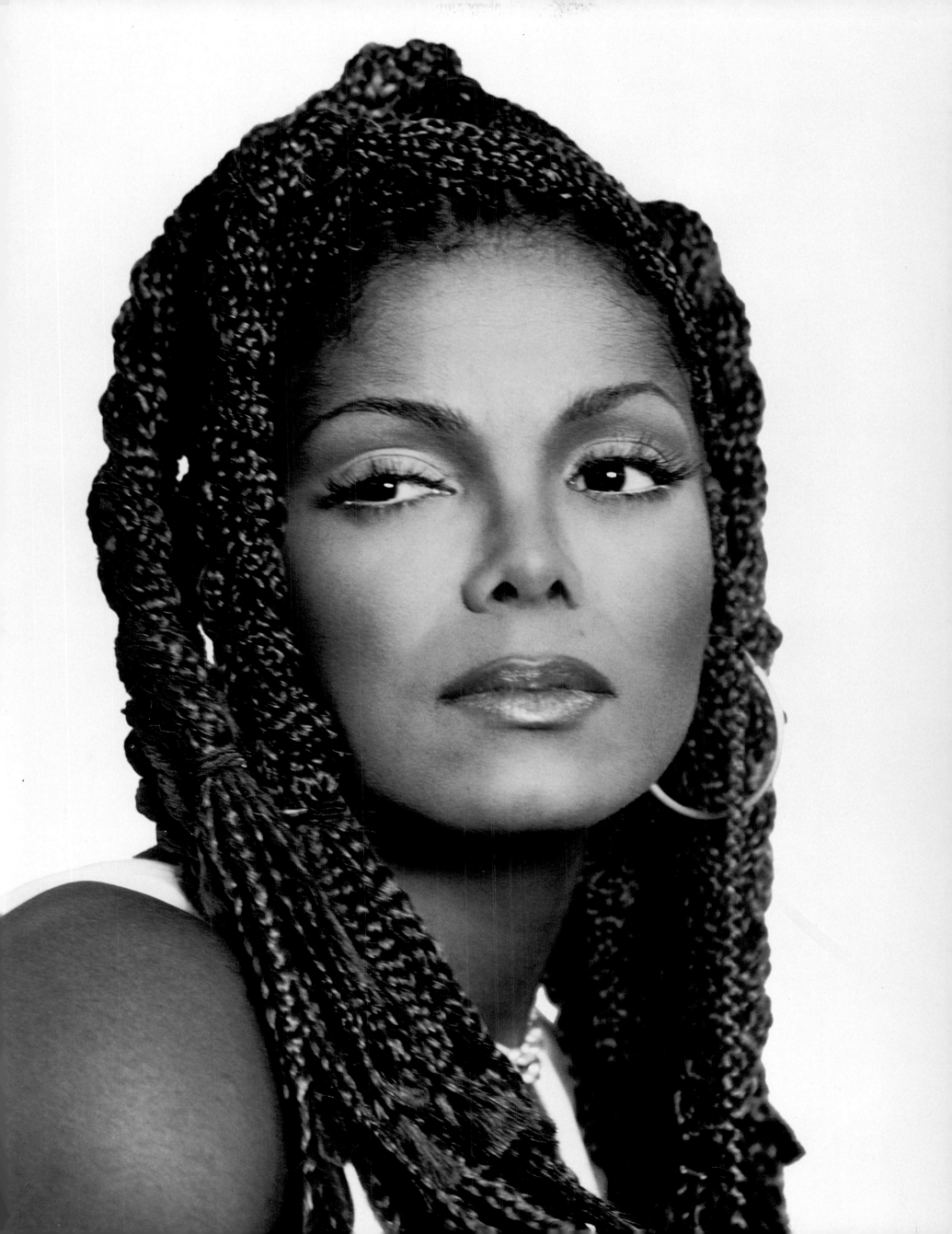

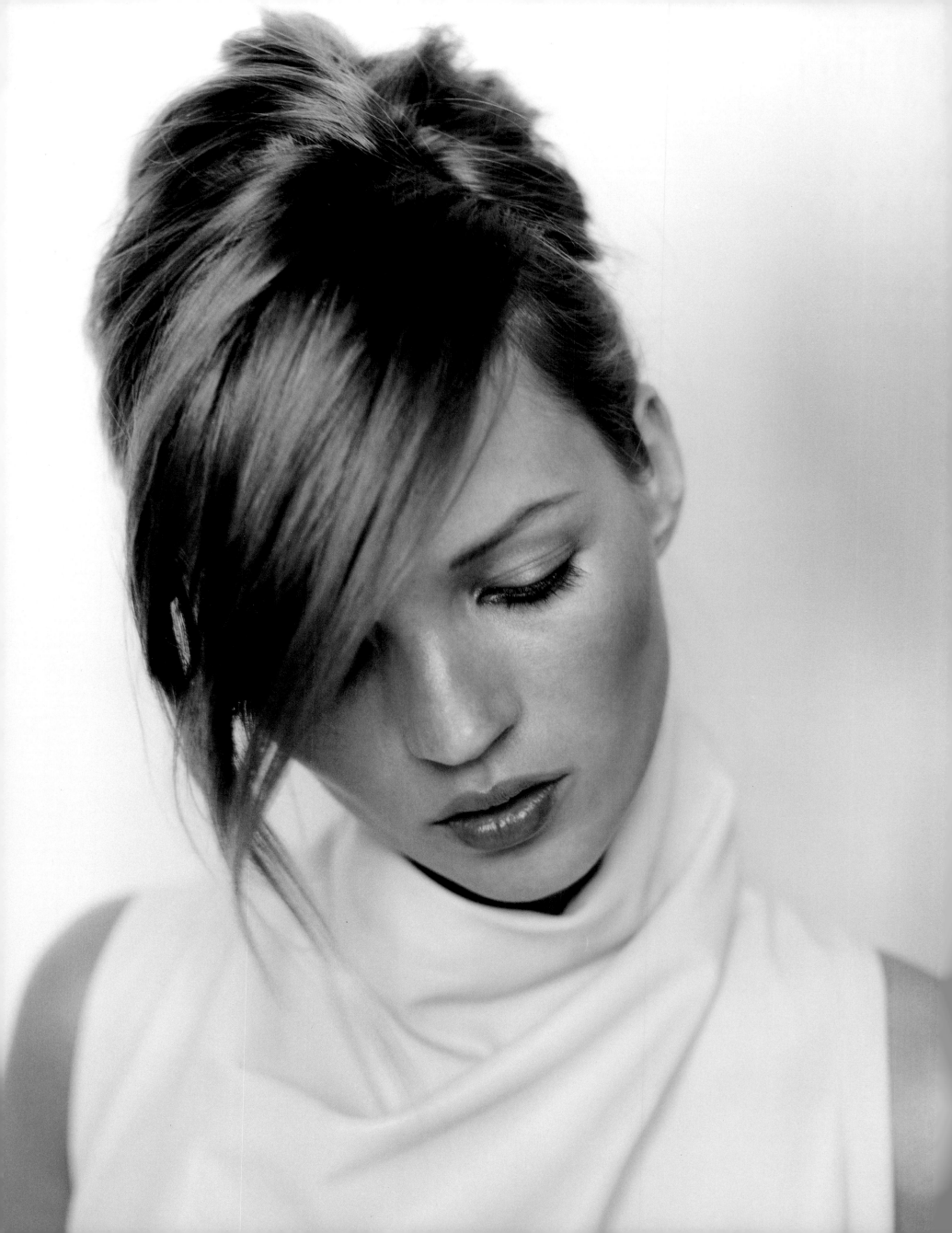

Preface

Liz Tilberis

When I started at British *Vogue* in the late 60s, it was a time of serious hair-styling: It was a fantasy time for very beautiful, posed, detailed, glittery, and exquisitely perfect creations. I noticed right away that the *coolest* guy on our sittings – the one who people hung around, listened to, and worshipped – was the hairdresser. Everyone would wait for the hairdresser to act. The very first fashion sitting I did was with photographer Hans Feurer and hairstylist Jean Louis David. Didier Malige was assisting on the hair. That day marked the beginning of my 25-year friendship and work relationship with Didier. Looking back, it's fun to see that many who were assistants then are the main guys now. Both Didier and Sam McKnight grew up with me in London.

This was also the wonderful moment when hairstyling for sittings became a specialized art form and career path. No longer was the sitting's hair-stylist always the same guy who worked in a salon. (I say "guy" because there were very, very few women in those days – and there are remarkably few, even today.) This book is a celebration of the vision, talent, and influence of this modern breed of studio hairstylists. As the pictures attest, most of them have a keen awareness of the demands of the camera, the agenda of the fashion editor, and the psyche of the model.

All the great hairdressers – people like Julien, Orlando, Sam, Didier – are extremely focused and patient. They, probably more than any others present at a sitting, are the diplomats who manage to bring together disparate personalities and ideas into a cohesive whole. Some members of this group have never even worked in a salon, never done cuts or blow-drys for commercial trade; others, notably Frederic Fekkai and John Sahag, balance a booming salon business with studio work.

Kate Moss, with hair styled by Orlando Pita, photographed by Mario Testino for *Harper's Bazaar. Courtesy Harper's Bazaar*

Sam cut my hair for many years and now Didier does it. Yet when someone asks me who my hairstylist is, I always hesitate to answer since it's virtually impossible to book an appointment with Didier. Normally, I recommend Frederic's salon in New York, as that is the salon with which Didier is associated. But given that sitting stylists don't often work in salons, there's often an element of confusion for women who set out to find the hairdressers whose work they admire in fashion magazines.

The pictures in this book chronicle the refinement of the art of studio hairdressing over the past two decades. In the 90s, studio hairstylists are asked to live in two completely different creative worlds. In some situations, they are asked to do realistic and beautiful hair, whether it's fresh and natural or tousled and sexy. Today, that typically means conservative and minimally styled hair, because that's where fashion is and what women want. In other situations, the hairstylist must offer serious comment on the way hair is going. They are asked to make a statement that is much more directional and detailed and often contains an element of fantasy.

Some people might dismiss the most outrageous of these looks as superfluous or out-of-touch. But I believe this sort of fantasy is necessary in order for women to dream. It's much the same with couture dresses. Few of us are able to afford a couture dress, but we like to dream about it. And that may inspire us to see ourselves in a whole new way.

When I was made the editor of British *Vogue*, my hair became my trademark. The straightness and the sleekness of my chin-length white bob was quite recognizable. (I was really covering a fat face!) Later, when I moved to America to re-launch *Harper's Bazaar*, my bob continued to serve me well. But when I had cancer and was about to start chemotherapy, Didier came to me and said, "Listen, the best thing to do is to cut it right now, very, very short, before you go in for the treatment." So we did cut it very short. Later, it did fall out in handfuls, which was very unpleasant. It is a superficial thing to say, but it is hurtful to know your hair is going to fall out. It is the most vulnerable place for women. It is a serious panic, because for an awful lot of us, our hair is our identity. But something positive did come out of the terrible. My hair began to grow back and, since I had lost weight, Didier suggested that I keep it short. And he's kept it short ever since, which is great. Sometimes it takes a lot of courage, but you must never be afraid to change your image.

All the hairstylists featured in this book have done a terrific job of

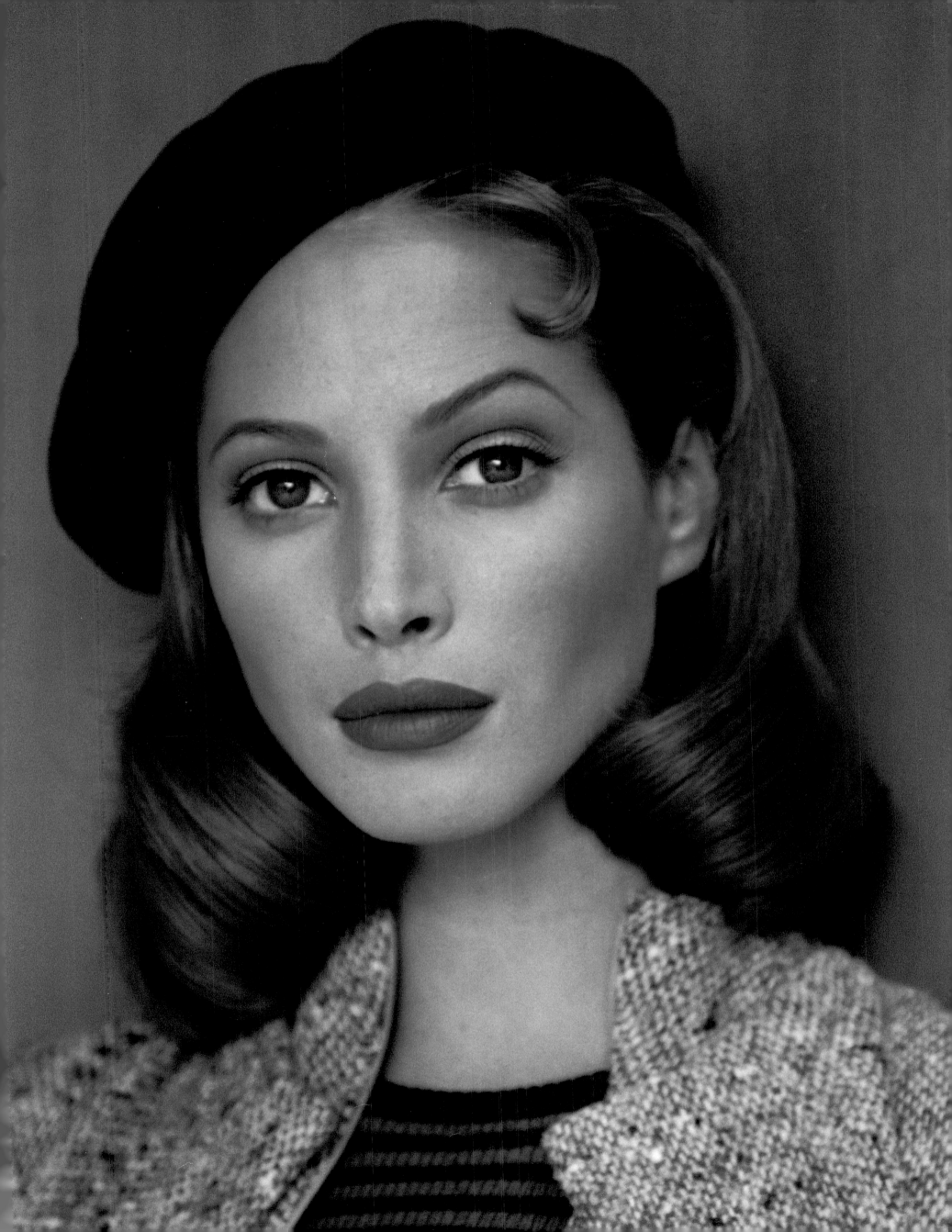

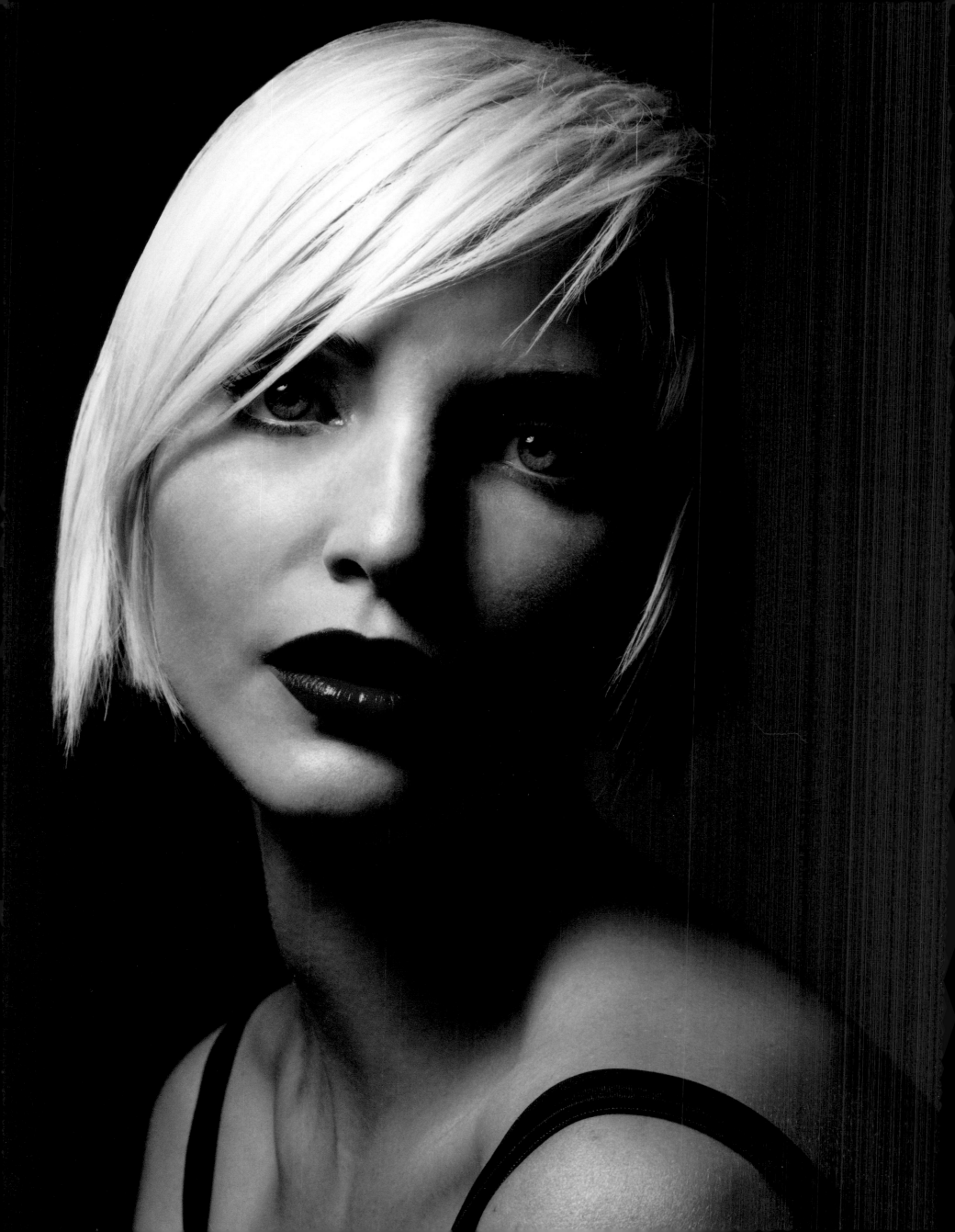

educating women in the modern thinking about hair. Thanks to them, women understand the basic concept of using what they've got naturally. Today, it's about wonderfully healthy hair, rather than hairdos. Rarely is there any of the back combing and setting and sleeping in rollers that I did in the 60s. So if you've got hair that can be corn rowed and it looks beautiful that way, put in fabulous plaits. If you just have straight hair that needs to be cut quite short, shop around for the perfect cut. If you want to wear your hair long, you'll need to learn how to look after it properly. There's been a tremendous education in hair, and with that education comes enormous freedom.

Women going forward into the next century have the luxury of a great deal of information, and styling and cutting talent, as well as amazingly sophisticated product technology. Most of this has come about through the work and vision of these stylists. I respect them tremendously.

I noticed right away that the *coolest* guy on our sittings – the one who people hung around, listened to, and worshipped – was the hairdresser. Everyone would wait for the hairdresser to act.

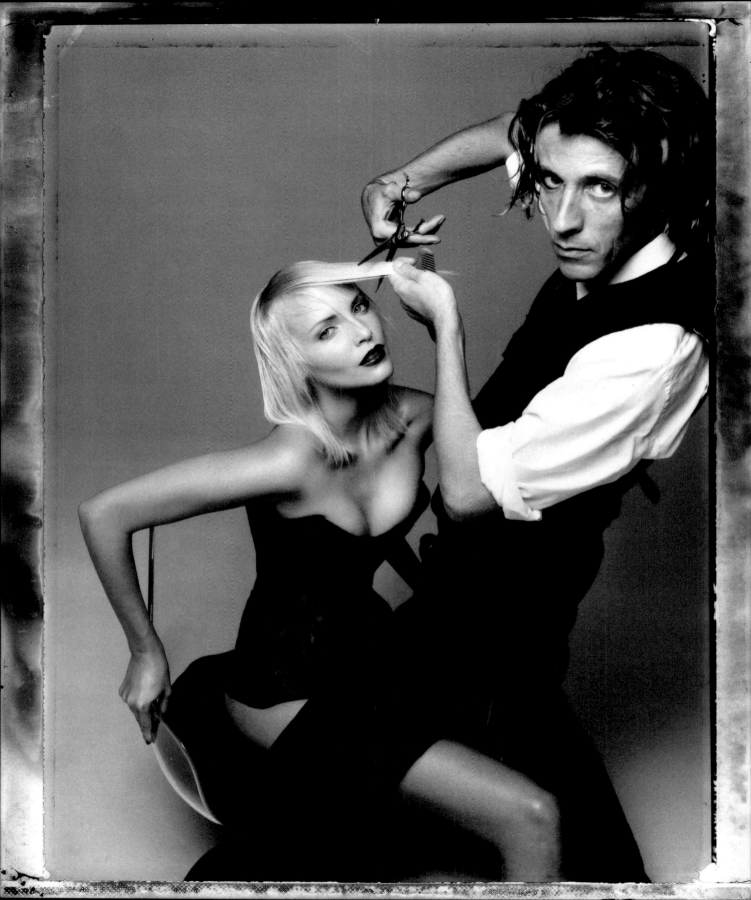

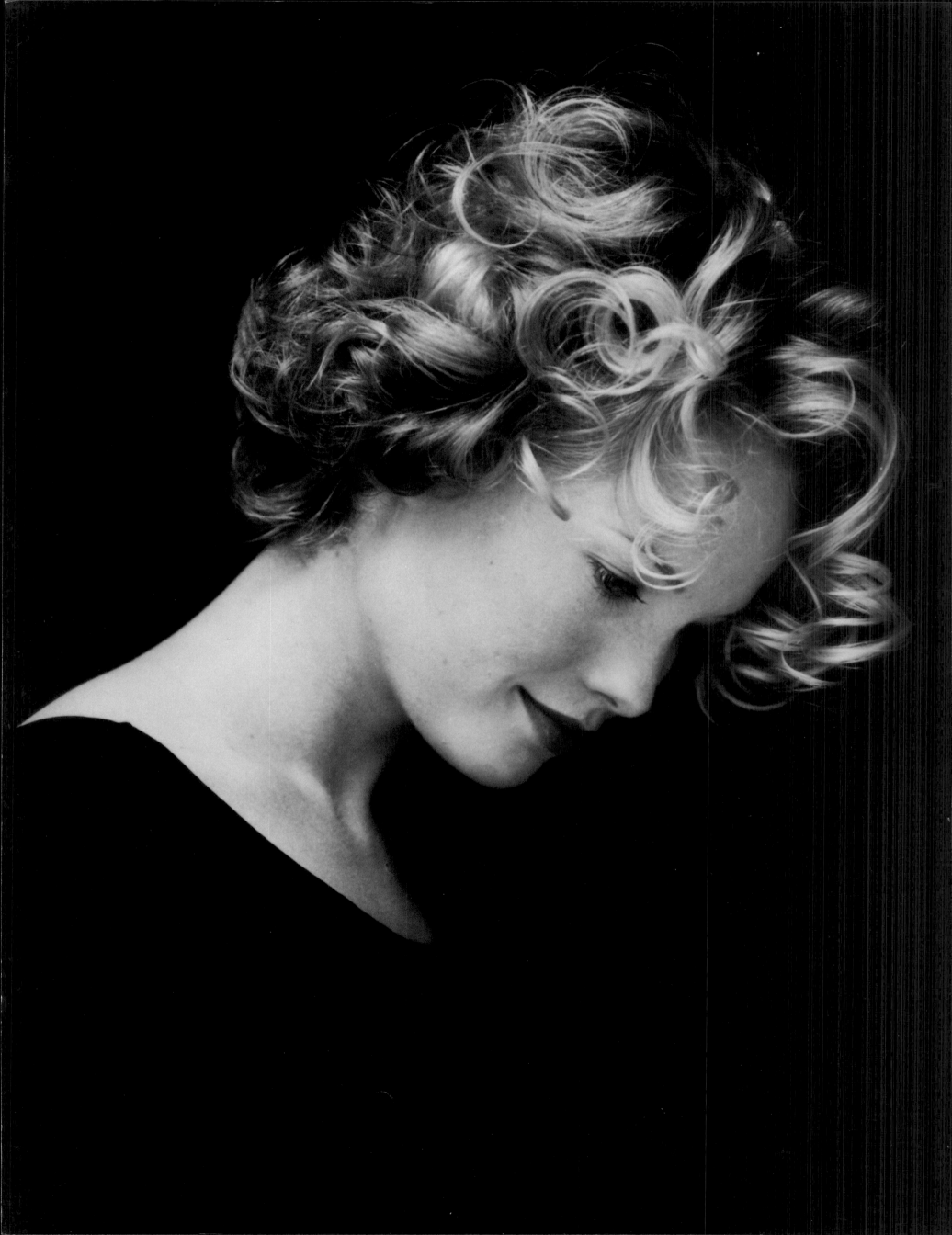

Hair Lines

A Brief History of Hair Style

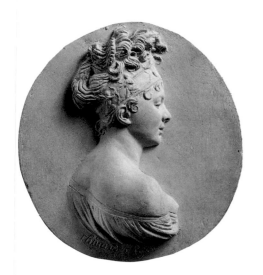

Portrait relief of Madame Juliette Récamier in terracotta, c. 1802, by Joseph Chinard. Private collection

Madame Juliette Récamier, one of the leading post-revolutionary style setters, is depicted here with an antique-inspired hairstyle. The elaborately curled and woven coiffure was considered quite simple after the sky-scraping hair constructions worn by aristocratic ladies before the French Revolution. Looking back to ancient Greece and Rome, women wore short hair, sometimes curled or waved with oil, held back by bands or ornaments as shown on ancient coins and portraits. The long ponytail caught up at the back of the head is most likely a hairpiece.

Hair has always been as much on women's minds as on their heads. How else to explain the enduring fascination of such tales as Delilah's betrayal of Samson, the wooing of Rapunzel, and the sacrifice of Jo's hair in *Little Women?* In "Goldilocks and the Three Bears," the heroine is even named for her hairtype. Hair is, after all, a woman's most identifying characteristic – for better or for worse, she will be categorized as a blonde, brunette, or redhead before ever being labeled as clever or dull. According to the great 20th-century arbiter of taste, Diana Vreeland, a woman's style starts with hair and moves downward to the clothes.

Hair, with its light-catching radiance, links us to the angels, but in its similarity to fur, unites us with the beasts. Hair is, in fact, an evolutionary hangover – we could certainly survive quite adequately without our hirsute head coverings. Maybe that is why aliens of higher intelligence in sci-fi movies are so often portrayed as bald. For many millennia now, hair has been primarily ornamental or symbolic – of age, rank, politics (the Clintons' haircuts work against their credibility), or sexual availability (porn stars' hair is usually as loose as their morals). Hair inspires so many decorative and metaphorical possibilities because it is the only truly malleable, transformable part of the body. How easy it is to alter a hairstyle – how difficult to control the contours of face or figure.

In virtually all cultures, women (financial and social position permitting) have called upon some kind of expert to help them dress their hair. A flair with hair was not exactly a ticket to social ascension, however. In ancient Rome, the

Hair styled by Bruno Pittini, photographed by Adel Awad for *Jacques Dessange Collection: A Forty-Year Retrospective.*
Hair color by L'Oréal Technique Professionnelle. © Jacques Dessange

ornatrix, a female specially trained in the art of hair arranging, created the coifs of highborn ladies – who when displeased with the outcome beat their attendant with a hand mirror. (Today ladies can leave the looking glass on the vanity and reach for the telephone instead; in Birmingham, England, there is a lawyer who specializes in hair malpractice.)

In slaveless societies, ladies' maids handled their mistresses' tresses. In some periods this could be a fairly simple undertaking – during the Middle Ages, when hair was considered too erotically charged, it was shaved at the brow and concealed beneath an elaborate, inviolable headdress, a version of which is still worn today by some nuns. (Early in her career as a Carmelite Sister, St. Teresa of Avila discovered the versatility of her wimple: she used it to crimp her hair.) Nor was much skill required during the high Victorian mid-19th century when respectable women wore severe (and, usually, severely unflattering) ear-covering chignons, center parted, and stiff, blinder-like bonnets. Talk about fashion slavery!

The hairdresser as we know him today – a skilled, respected, and independent professional who practices his art on more than one woman – emerged from the courts of the 17th century when coiffure became ostentatiously, and fantastically, intricate. In Spain, King Philip IV conferred the same rank on his court barber as on Diego Velázquez, his court painter. Although the Catholic Church threatened to excommunicate any woman who dared let a man coif her hair, males dominated the field then as now. The profession seems, in fact, to have leapt into being fully formed, every stereotype firmly in place. Imperious, temperamental, gossipy, doted on by the ladies, and often addressed by first name only, the hairdresser cliché shows up not only in *ancien régime* accounts of Versailles, but also in antebellum recollections of New York. In this New World outpost, a certain Monsieur Martelle, "a dainty half-Spanish or French octoroon endowed with exquisite taste, a ready wit, and saucy tongue," one contemporary noted, captivated every fashionable head. Likewise, Legros de Rumigny dictated hair modes to women in pre-revolutionary France. This enterprising former cook (maybe this is why hairdos of the period resembled pastries) founded an academy of coiffures, publicized his designs on miniature hairdo dolls, and published a textbook, all under the name "Legros." A hairdresser's monopoly could be so absolute that on busy occasions, such as New Year's Day in New York, he would fix the hair of less prestigious clients the evening before, leaving them to sit up all night so as not to spoil Monsieur's masterpiece.

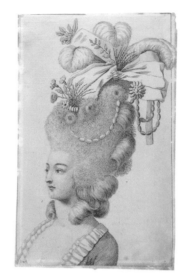

Print, c. 1770, from collection of Miriam and Ira D. Wallach Division of Art, Prints and Photographs, The New York Public Library, Astor, Lenox and Tilden Foundations

A tall, beribboned coiffure styled when hair often reached a height of three feet, sometimes higher when adorned with feather plumes. A woman's own hair was used as the anchor for horsehair pads, which were wire-framework hairpieces coated with bear's grease or lard. The arrangement was heavily adorned with frou-frou – sometimes the decoration was thematic or allegorical – and finally powdered with wheat flour.

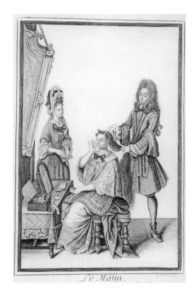

French engraving, late 17th century. Courtesy Stubbs Books and Prints, New York

An engraving showing the hairdresser's morning visit. Court ladies also set each other's hair in the evening. Such hairdressing sessions were social activities that provided a relaxing, informal break from rigid and stifling court etiquette.

Nadja Auermann, with hair styled by Julien d'Ys, photographed by Karl Lagerfeld for Karl Lagerfeld

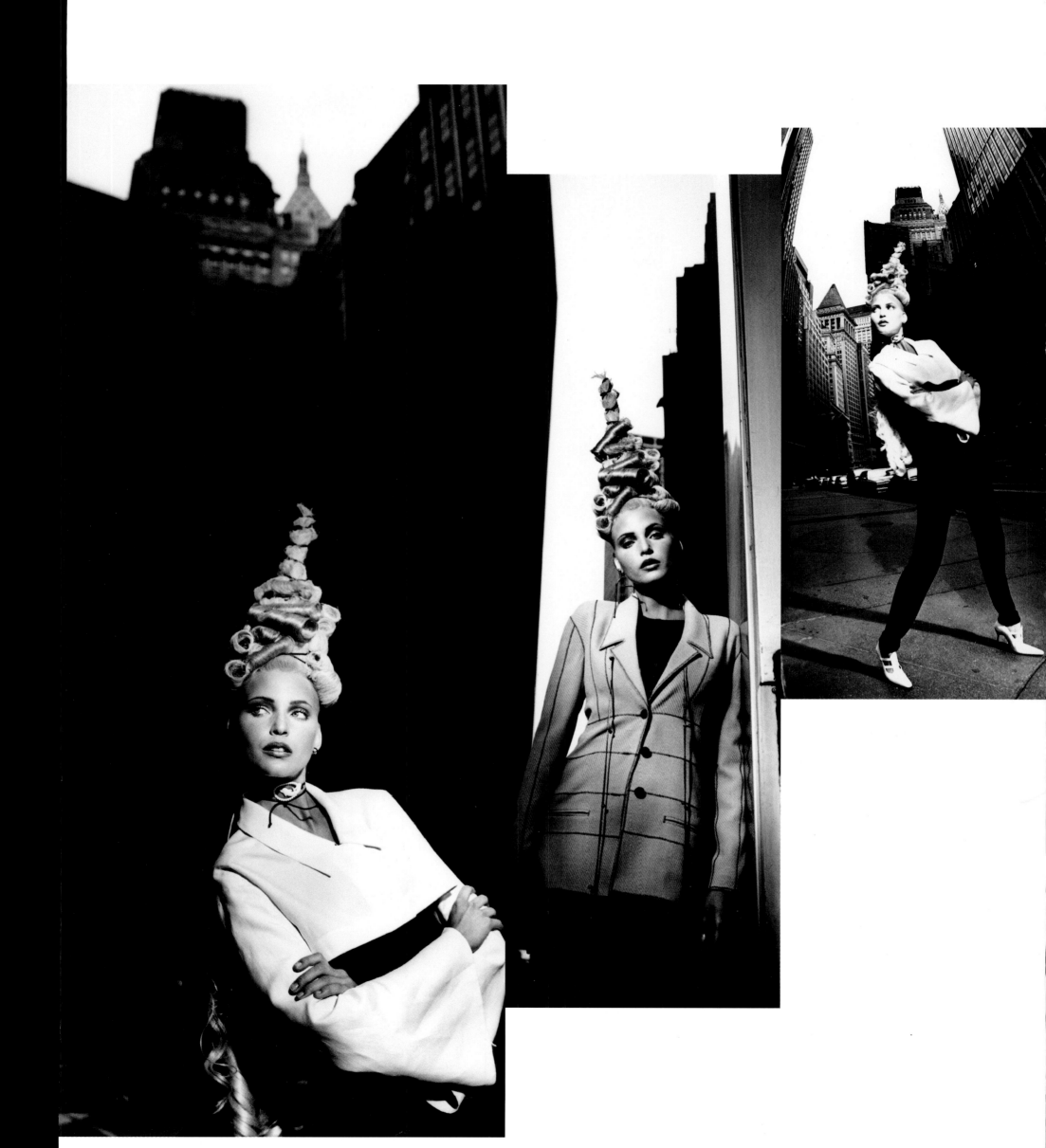

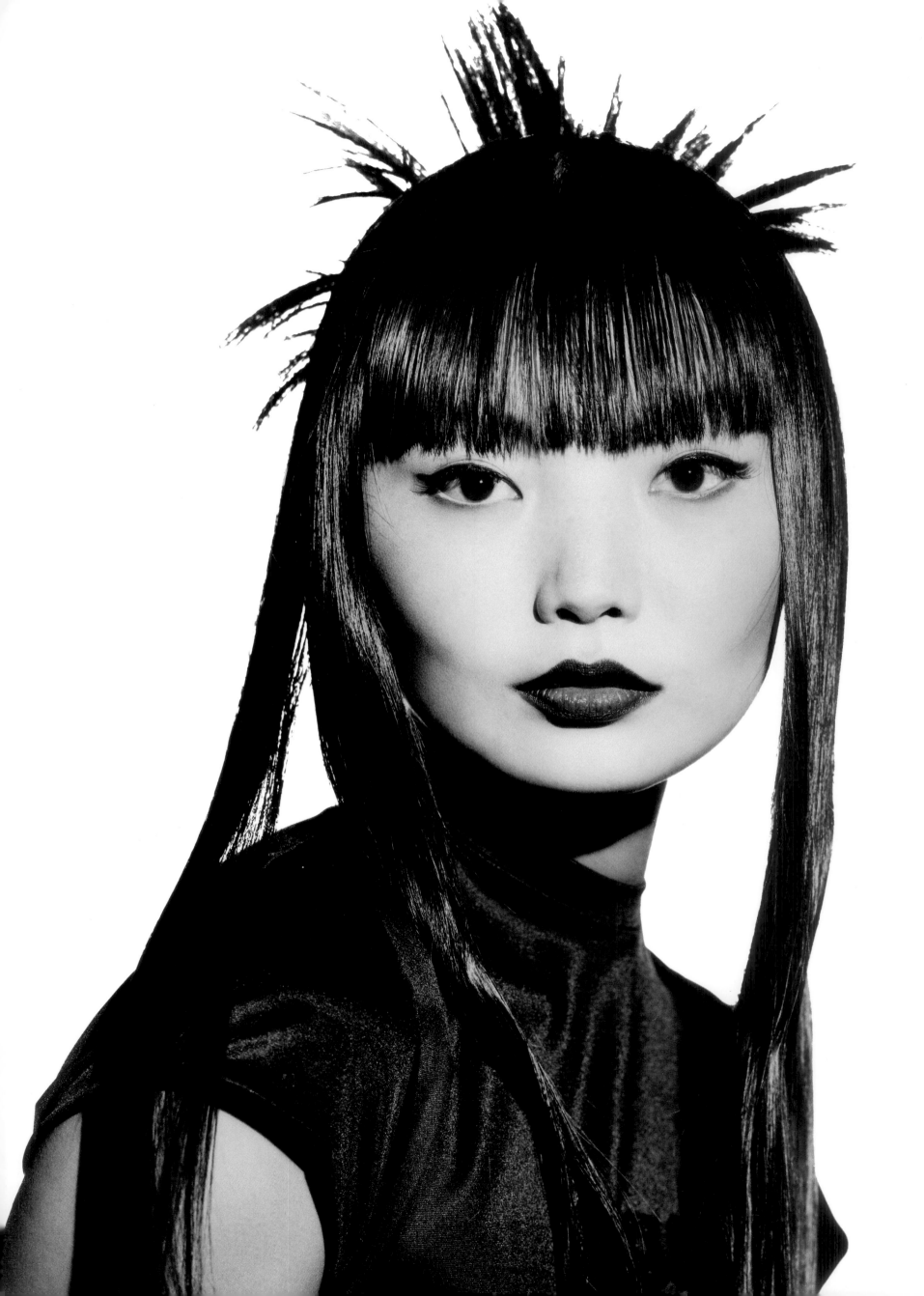

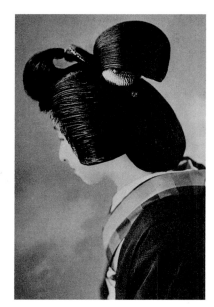

Photograph, 1937. Private collection

This style originally flourished in the 17th and 18th centuries and became recognized as traditional Japanese hairstyling. The technique involved padding the hair and shaping it with a fat-based pomade, similar to the technique used by the European court hairdressers of the day.

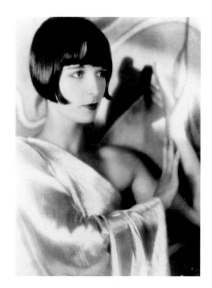

Louise Brooks. Still from the MGM Collection, used by permission of Turner Entertainment Co.

If, historically, hairdressers have had a reputation for being difficult, consider some of their frustrations. Not quite an artist, and no longer a servant, a confidant of the ladies, but not a social equal, they were routinely suspected of either corrupting women or reviling them. No wonder the profession has attracted such formidable personalities! Who could be more flamboyantly eccentric than the great Antoine (the Picasso of hair, he introduced the bob at the same moment that the modernist painter invented Cubism) — except, perhaps, his client Sarah Bernhardt. Both slept in coffins, although Antoine, the more fully 20th-century character, had his constructed of glass.

Antoine was one of several visionaries who ushered ideas about hair out of the Dark Ages and into the 20th century. Not until around 1890 had it even been considered healthy to wash one's hair — a vestige, most likely, of the pagan superstition that water disturbed the spirit guarding the head. Throughout the centuries, recipes for hair tonics read like formulas for witch's brew. In the Middle Ages, leech skins were a recommended scalp nourisher. In 18th-century England, hog lard was extolled as a superior cleanser for children's hair. Arsenic and lead were stirred into Renaissance bleaching potions. Marie Antoinette's hair glop consisted mostly of grease, flour, and glue. Until this century, haircutting techniques were equally primitive. In fact, Victorian women were so loathe to give up any of their precious strands, they wove their hair clippings into elaborate jewelry, frames, and other mementos. Leila Calhoon has collected 1,000 such specimens — including an 1852 floral tapestry crafted from the hair of 156 members of a single family — and installed them in the Hair Museum, a division of her Independence College of Cosmetology.

Early 20th-century innovations, such as the permanent wave machine, the dryer, and reliable bleaches, finally coaxed women, in reversal of the traditional custom, out of their boudoir and into the hairdresser's chair — now set up in publicly accessible shops. These establishments sought to appease lingering middle-class anxieties about the propriety of dressing hair outside the home by assuming the names of tony private rooms — e.g., the "salon" or the "parlor" — and by adopting reassuringly pseudo-aristocratic "Louis Quelque chose" decor.

Increasingly democratized by movies and mass media, hair fashions in recent decades have become based more on the cut than on setting or arranging. Though women's trips to the "beauty parlor" may be less frequent than a generation ago, the hairdresser is not about to abdicate his hydraulic throne.

Irina Pantaeva, with hair styled by John Sahag, photographed by Albert Watson

No refinement in at-home perm or coloring kits, no improvements in do-it-yourself gels and rollers, can replace the camaraderie, intimacy, and prowess of the professional hairstylist. And no scientific breakthrough is ever likely to enable a woman to guide a pair of scissors dextrously across the nape of her neck.

Today — more than a hundred years after the inauguration of modern hair technology — top stylists have become, along with supermodels, photographers, and designers, media sensations in their own right. This trend, like so many others, can probably be traced to Vidal Sassoon, whose legendary career as cut-and-blow pioneer and haircare entrepreneur has inspired two books and a museum retrospective. Perhaps the fame of clients has finally rubbed off on the hairstylist — along with a bit of dye and spray. Not to mention that in the late 20th century, when social and professional hierarchies of all kinds are collapsing, the distinction between the applied art of hair design and the fine arts (painting and sculpture) is becoming more blurred. In accordance with this elevated stature, a new breed of stylist has emerged — the session man who works only on celebrities' and supermodels' hair for magazine shoots or ad campaigns, never in a salon.

This book pays homage to today's international hair stars, a pantheon of contemporary masters whose work is featured regularly in every authoritative fashion publication, trend-setting music video, and influential ad campaign — as well as on ultra-fashionable heads the world over. Up-and-coming and well-established, avant-garde and classical, studio stylists and salon owners, are artists whose medium happens to be hair. Out of its tangled chaos, they create order and beauty, however short-lived. As Alexandre, the great Parisian coiffeur who shaped the locks (and the destiny) of Jacqueline Kennedy Onassis and Elizabeth Taylor, once wrote, hairstyling is "a desperate search for an eternal and fugitive beauty . . . the search for that which will last only for one day." This book, a portable gallery of the best work of the most eminent stylists, will finally give more permanence to their evanescent art.

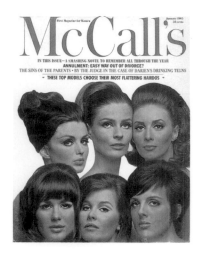

Photograph by Melvin Sokolsky. Courtesy *McCall's*

In 1965, McCall's magazine published this cover featuring six top models in "their most flattering hairdos." Kenneth, the legendary hairstylist who created the styles on two of the models, noted in McCall's, "Every one of the models had her hair set under a dryer. None of them would have gone out of the house without her hair totally done, finished."

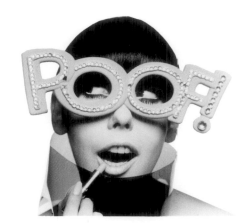

Peggy Moffatt, with hair styled by Vidal Sassoon, photographed by Neal Barr

Linda Evangelista, with hair styled by Michel Aleman for Frederic Fekkai, photographed by Gilles Bensimon for American *Elle*. Courtesy American *Elle*

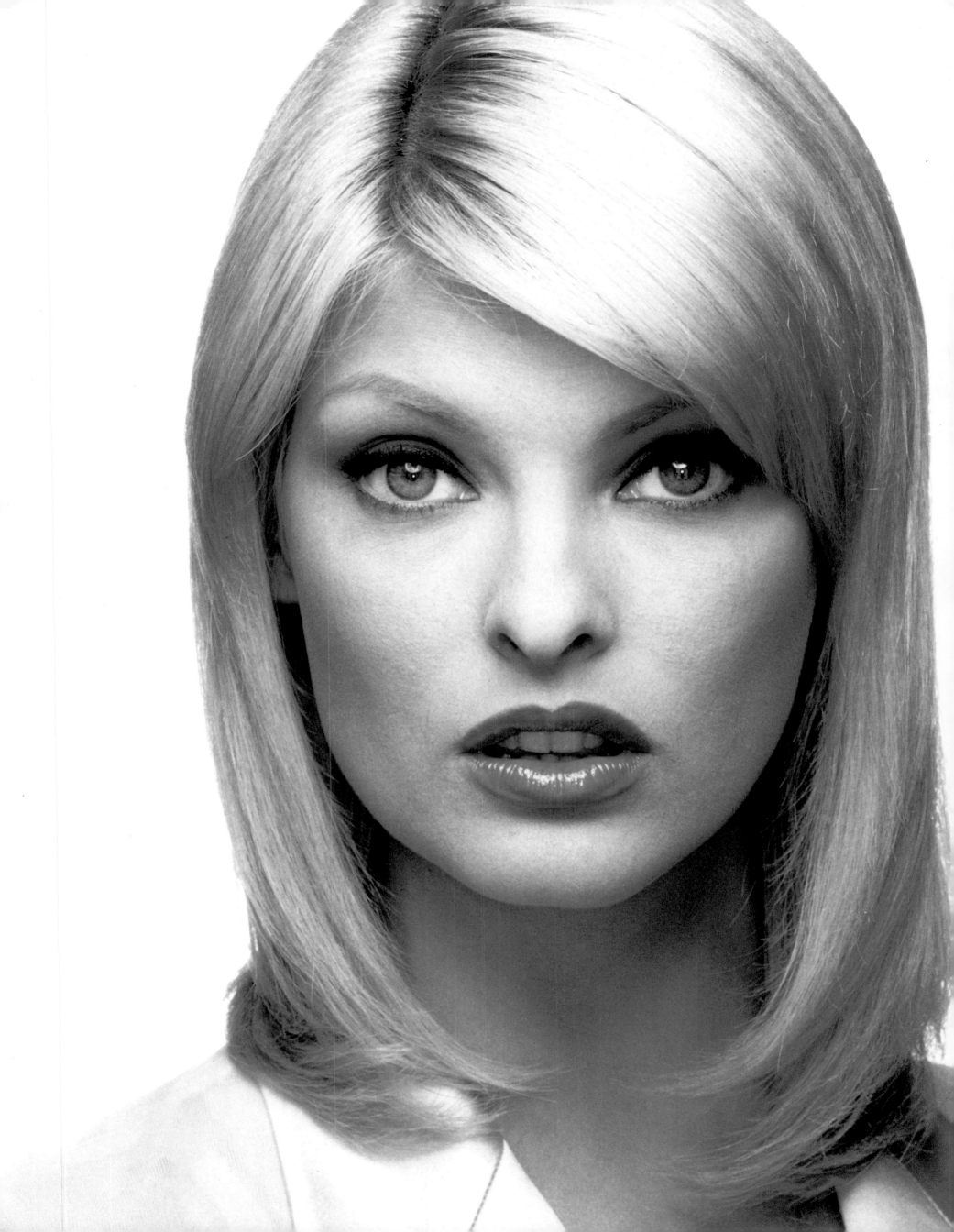

CHRISTIAAI
SFREDERICH
MTKNKSD
ESAMMCKM
ENORMAI
DOPITAJOI

Profile

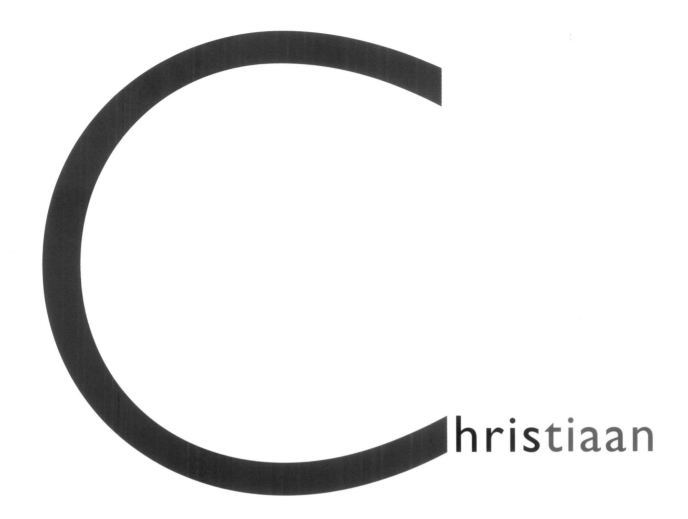

Christiaan

Philosopher of Hair

Christiaan is hairdressing's wild man – an unreconstructed hippie, anarchic sage, and all-around nonconformist. There is no question which door on the fifth floor of an undistinguished building in a gritty West Side neighborhood belongs to the hairstylist Christiaan. One is pristine and clearly indicated with the letter "B." The other is battered, peeling, and illegibly marked. The man who answers the door (and to the incongruously pious name) is a tall, tousled soul bearing more than a passing resemblance to the actor Nick Nolte. His handsome face is as deeply weathered as a chunk of driftwood, and his matted hair (at least in the front) is colored a daffodil yellow. It is cut or, rather, torn into a style he calls "Dutch flaps." Two longish pieces flop like a mongrel's ears on either side of his head, while the back is shorn up to the level of his neck. Christiaan wears a colorfully ageless and androgynous outfit of a dandelion pullover, green, yellow, and blue striped pants, and white sneakers. A gentle, ragamuffin giant, he eases his large frame into a gilded armchair in his sunny living room, furnished with a combination of flea-market finds and gifts from friends. With its bohemian lack of pretension and its multitude of paintings – from an academic portrait of a smoking woman to a modern study of the Crucifixion – the space looks more like an artist's studio than the home of someone connected to the world of fashion.

"I have modeled myself after a painter or a writer," Christiaan says, pouring tea from a ceramic pot. "No office, no secretary, no boss." Marianna, his wife of 27 years, acts as his agent, and for nearly as long he's been without a salon affiliation. "It puts you on a different plane – makes you more of an equal to everyone. I'm an independent character in this world." A kind of philosopher of hair, Christiaan is obsessed with the substance and all its metaphorical possibilities. "I relate to hair," he says. "Not to clothes or fashion. Hair is on all of us. You

"GREENOUT"

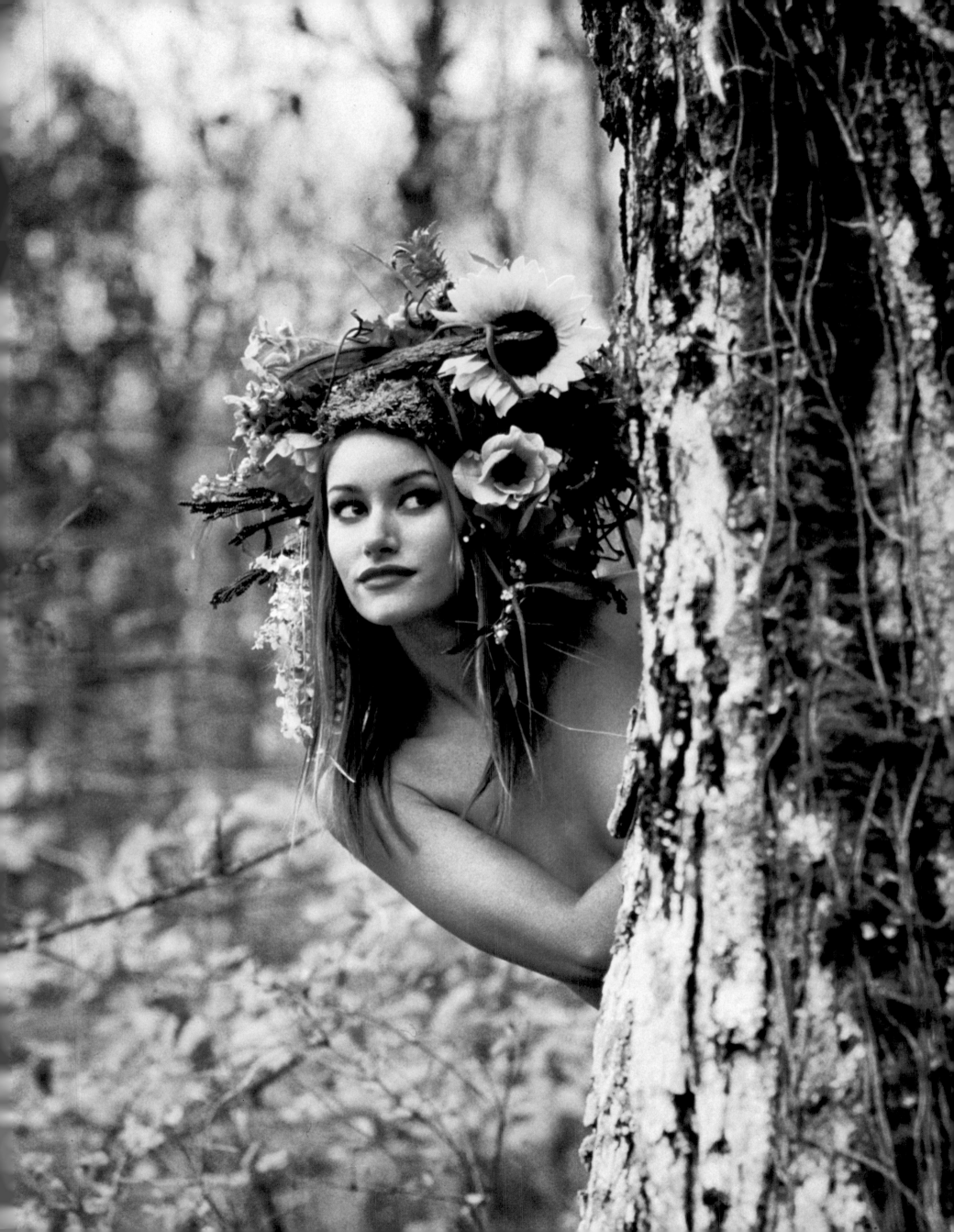

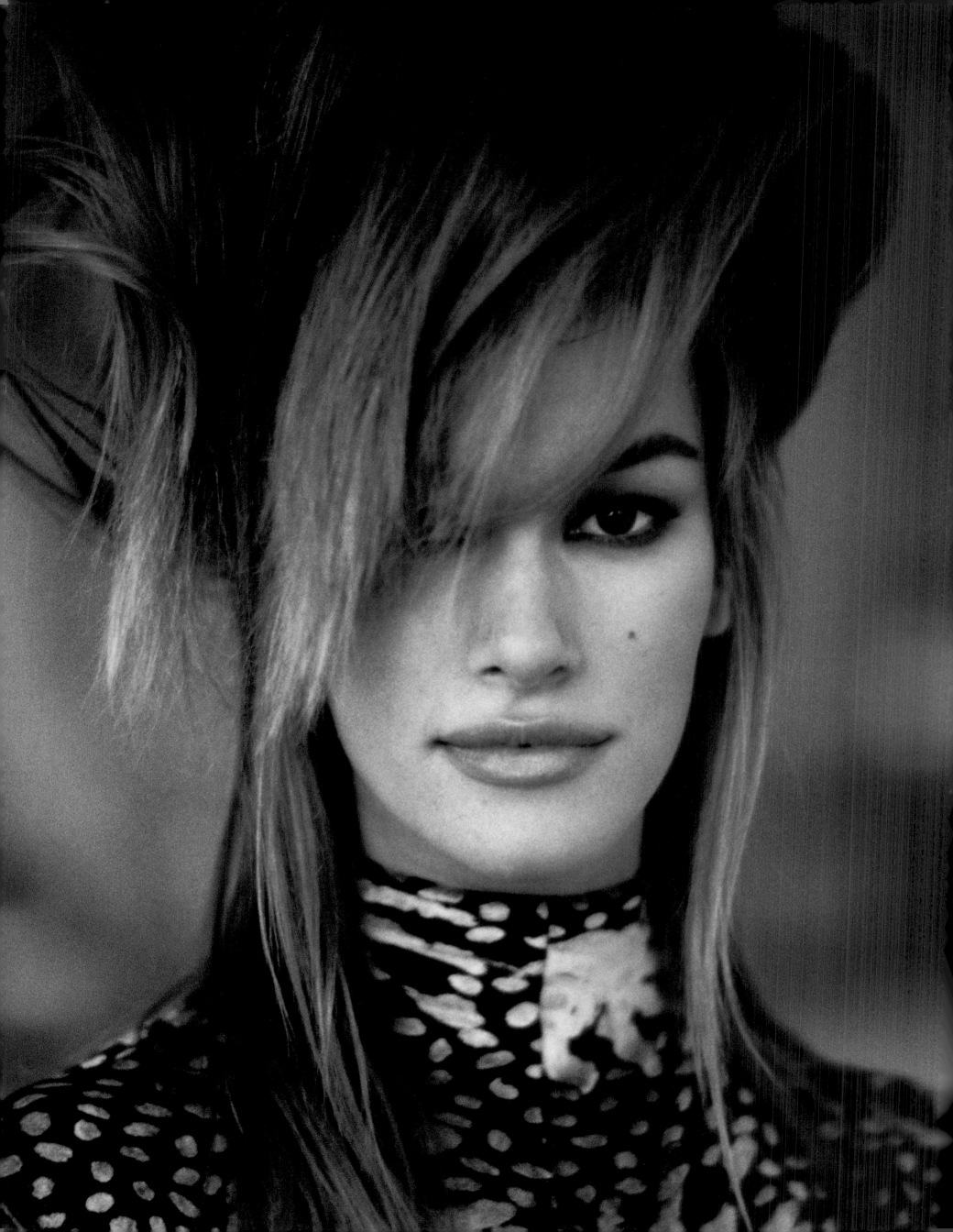

can't remove it like you do clothes. Since we all carry hair on us, we have to deal with it in some way. It is the only fluid part of our body – both in the time sense, because it grows and changes, and three-dimensionally too. For many years I contented myself with the idea that working with hair was like trying to control water. It can't be stopped. Hair always reverts to itself in the end. Now I'm focused on the process of doing it, not on the end result. It's none of my business what happens to hair after I've worked on it. It's too personal. I certainly don't like the idea of somebody saying [his voice rising mockingly], 'How do you like my Christiaan?' The hair does not belong to me."

What does belong to Christiaan are some very definite opinions about people taking control of the look of their own heads. "In the end, it's how you *think* about your hair, not how it looks, that counts. You should never hate your hair, or worry, 'Do I look good?' I'm opposed to the idea of loading up responsibilities. You shouldn't, for example, worry about roots – lately this idea is becoming more acceptable. Perms are always a dead end. Whatever you do with your hair, it should bring you peace and happiness, from the inside out. I also encourage people to cut their own hair. I tell my two boys – they're 13 and 16 – to cut it themselves. And I don't cut my wife's hair." Having once gone ten years without shampooing, he is also somewhat skeptical of commercial cleansers. "Water alone is really sufficient," he advises. He did, however, revert to sudsing when he started building – with-

out aid of architects or contractors – his family's country house in Water Mill, Long Island. "I was getting caked with mud."

The inventor of the buzz cut, Christiaan is also an impassioned advocate of shaving the head, a practice he began in 1984 on the model Bonnie Berman. "We were coming out of a period when hair was so natural, loose, and long it got boring. So I picked up the razor. With this recent return to glamour – which I think has set hair back a whole generation – I'm into shaving everyone again. Every so often I shave my own head. I really love bald heads. In the end, ten generations from now, we'll all be bald. Hair is disposable, a useless leftover. Sure, we still have some of it here and there," he says, slapping under his arm, and pointing to his groin, "just to keep the drips from going down our shirtsleeves and pants. But baldness is at least 50 times more prevalent today than when I was growing up."

Another of Christiaan's attempts to subvert hairdressing orthodoxies is the "digit" cut, an anti-precision approach that liberates the stylist from the comb – "more of a guerrilla tactic," he says, than a technique. He wets the hair and then inserts the scissors "like a pencil" at random spots in the hair, snipping it into a succession of "pluses and minuses," or into negative and positive thickets of hair. This peculiar practice results in short, choppy ripples, as if the hair has been whipped up by a strong wind. He recently tried out the digit cut on an "Asian neighbor girl. During the session she felt no sensation but her cut hair drifting down –

Hairstory

STYLIST: *Christiaan*
SALON ADDRESS: *None*
PLACE OF BIRTH: *Bovenkarspel, Holland*
FIRST JOB: *Age 12, cutting hair in his father's barber shop*
TRADEMARKS: *Metaphysical approach to hair and hairstyling; Nonconformity; Buzz cuts; Not accepting money from private clients; Flattop fades; "Digit" cuts*

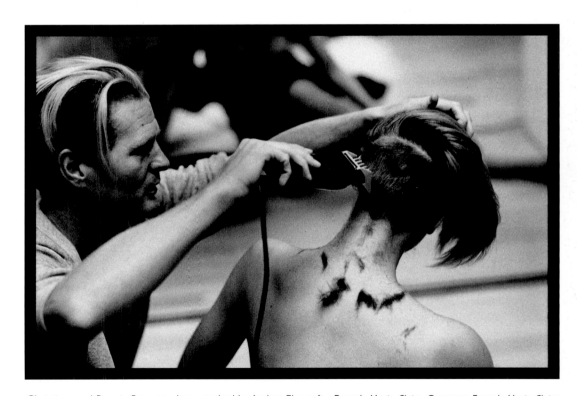

Christiaan and Bonnie Berman, photographed by Arthur Elgort for French *Marie Claire*. Courtesy French *Marie Claire*
"BUZZHEDD"

Susan Holmes, photographed by Arthur Elgort for Italian *Vogue*. Courtesy Italian *Vogue*

'FIGERME'

no comb touched her head. She was happy. The digit cut is quite possible if you know what you're doing."

Some time ago, Christiaan performed another successful experiment on a neighbor – Grace Jones, whom he had known since her modeling days. "Our apartment windows faced each other, and one night, after she had just broken up with her boyfriend, she screamed out the window, 'I want you to take it all off!' So I gave her a flattop – which was then copied by Carl Lewis and everybody else." Christiaan takes his scissors wherever he goes, giving cuts in bars and on sidewalks around the world. "I never charge. I don't like taking personal money – only corporate money." Recently he was in Lower Manhattan's Bowery Bar, where a fellow patron yelled out to him, "'Hey, you! You cut my hair at the Carlton Hotel in Cannes!' So I pulled out my scissors and gave him another haircut."

Having earned plenty of "corporate money" in his day – at some point he's worked for practically every major account – he can well afford his generosity. The commission currently occupying him is the hairstyling for Cleveland's new Rock and Roll Hall of Fame. "I'm doing the heads for Elvis, Axl Rose, Sly Stone, Jimi Hendrix. It's challenging because I'm supposed to find a generic look for each star, not one that is necessarily historically accurate to a certain period in their lives. I wanted to do Sly Stone as he looked at Woodstock, but instead he's getting a huge Afro. Usually I hate anything retro, but this is a little different. It's my favorite commercial assignment." Stephen Sprouse, the neopunk designer whose fashion shows Christiaan has always done ("He's a crucial individual in my life," says Sprouse), is the curator of the costumes and I. M. Pei, the architect of the building.

Though the Hall of Fame project involves dressing wigs, Christiaan prefers live hair. "I'd also rather not use extensions." Instead, to achieve unusual effects, he concocts new processes, such as "applying needle and thread to the hair." For a recent Liza Bruce show, he wove threads from hairline to crown, which left the front of the model's hair flattened as if by a headband, and the back hanging freely. He has also tried sewing into the strands a kind of hairnet, through which he pulls out clumps of hair, creating a variety of forms and textures on the head. To mold hair into gravity-defying shapes, he has also fortified it with thin, pliable wires. "Everything I do has to go up quickly, and then come down

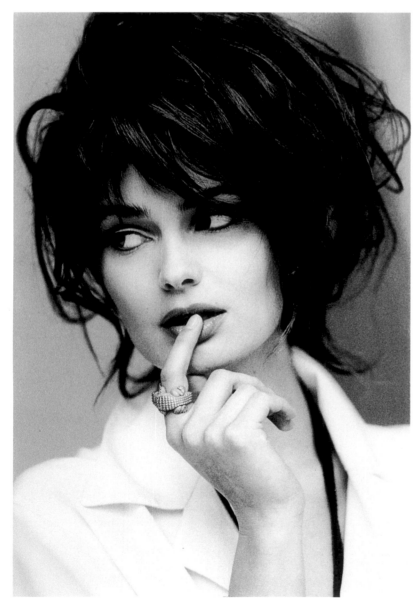

Paulina Porizkova, photographed by Arthur Elgort for French *Vogue*. Courtesy French *Vogue*

"FANCYMOI"

Claudia Schiffer, photographed by Arthur Elgort for American *Vogue*. Courtesy American *Vogue* ©The Condé Nast Publications Inc.

"PINMEUP"

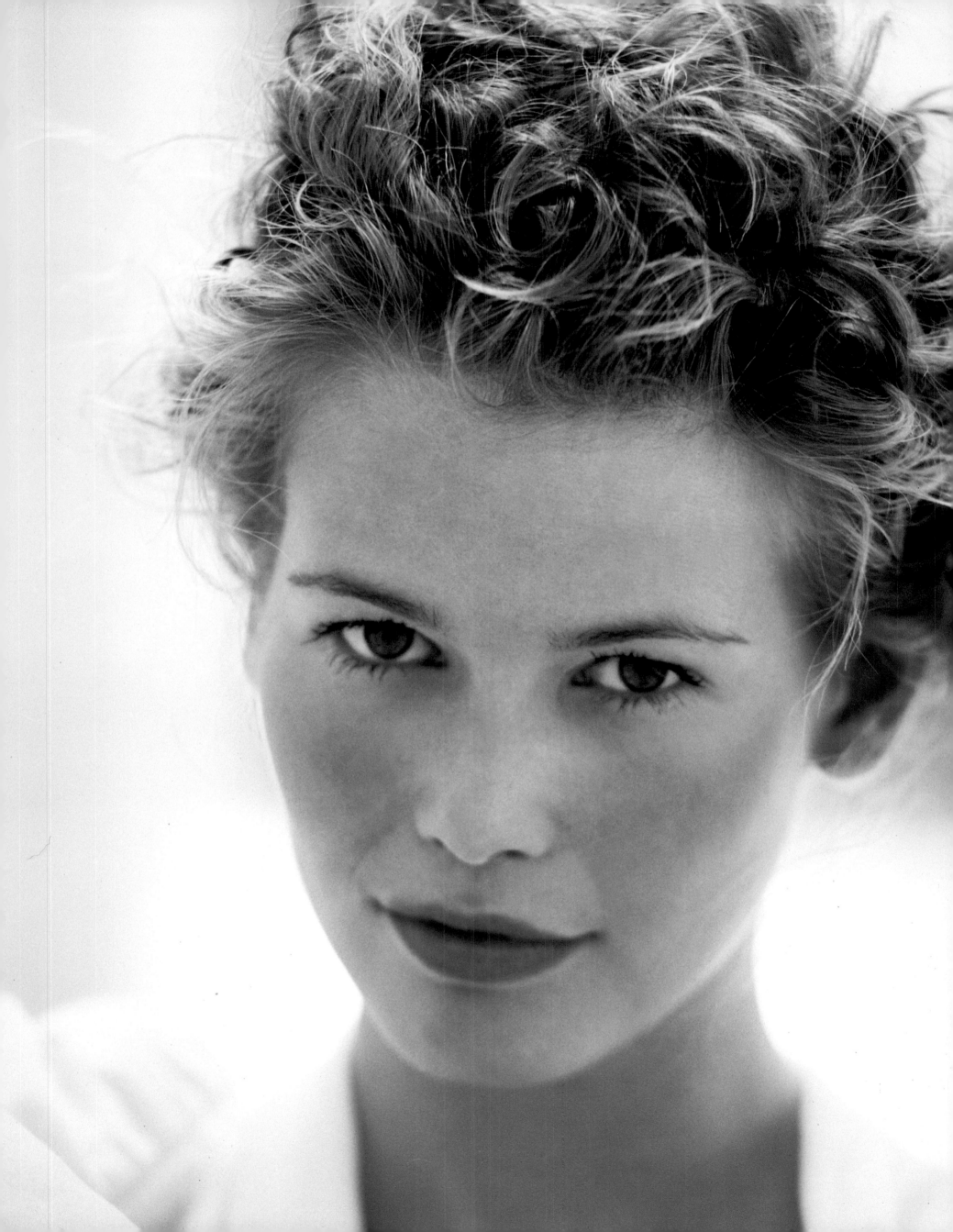

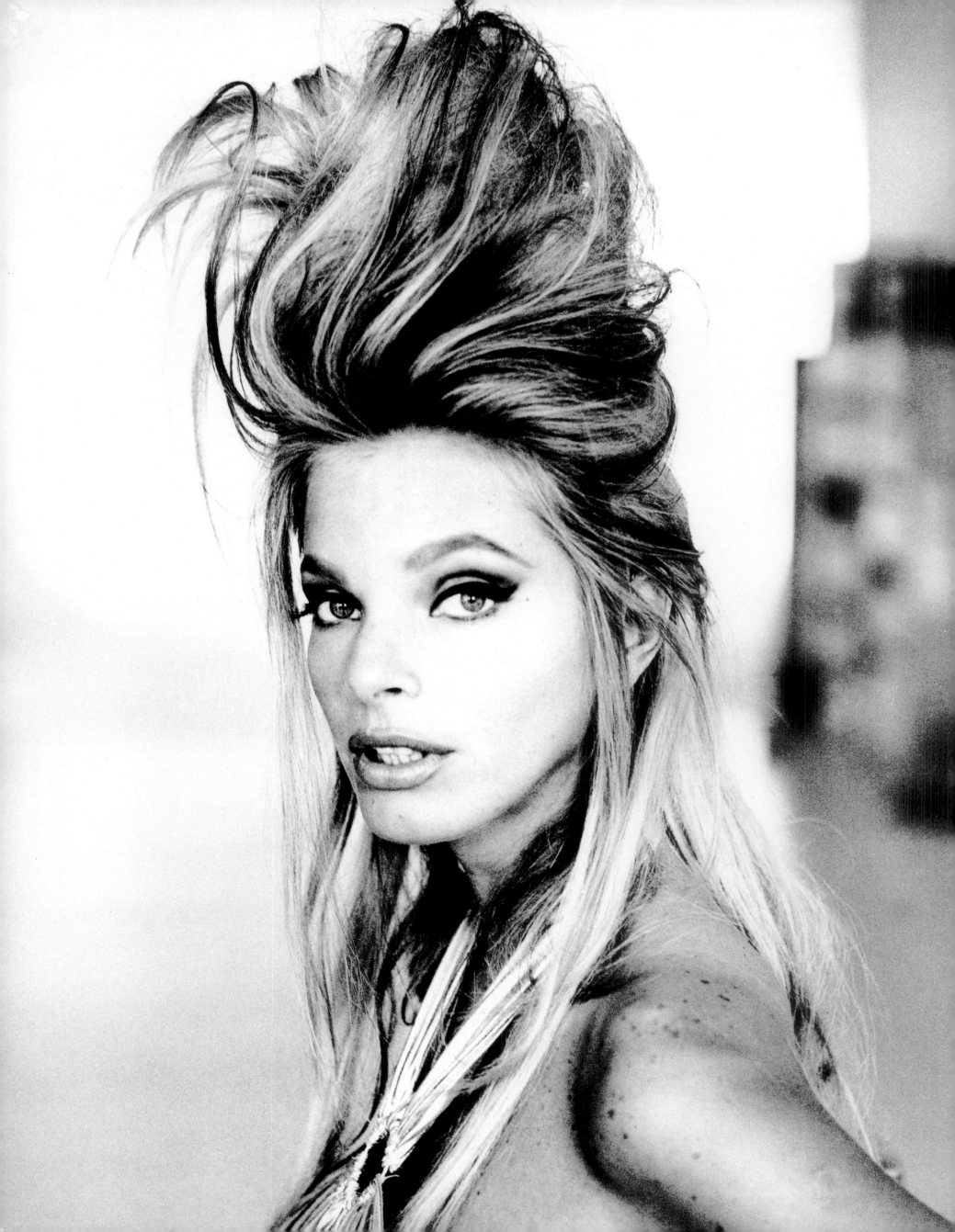

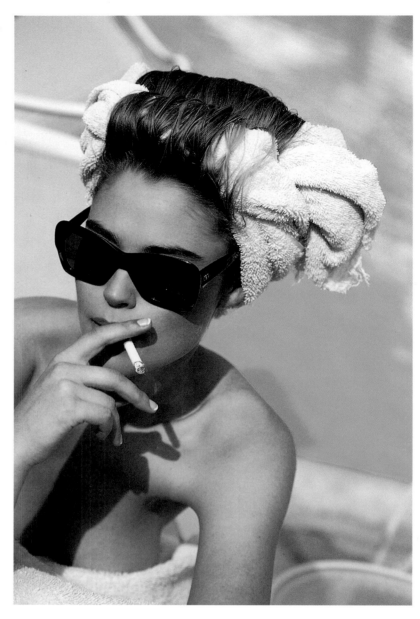

easily," he insists. "Even if I do a simple chignon. The days when I would do a chignon secured with 62 bobby pins are over. If what I'm doing hurts the girl, then I'm doing something wrong."

Christiaan has been evolving his quirky tonsorial wisdom over a period of 40 years. Born in the tulip-farming village of Bovenkarspel, Holland, on September 15, 1945, he was the oldest of the local barber's 12 children. At 12, he began working in his father's shop, where he absorbed such fundamental lessons as the importance of touch. "How you touch a person's head affects how you make them feel. There's no such thing as an ugly touch and beautiful results. If my father found me handling one of his customer's heads too roughly, he would strike my hand with a comb." Drafted at 18, he selected the Marines for the opportunity to travel. Stationed in Curaçao and Aruba, he trained as a demolitions expert and "sometime flame thrower. But I was cutting everyone's hair. I was a fanatic." Word of this scissors-crazed soldier reached Aruba's American compound, where the families employed by the island's Esso refinery resided. He became the favorite of a certain Mrs. Kurt Weill, wife of the oil refinery's president — not the wife of the illustrious German composer of *Threepenny Opera* fame. One day Mrs. Weill spotted a photograph

of then *Glamour* Editor-in-Chief Amy Green. Mistaking her for an ex-classmate, she dispatched a letter recommending Christiaan and his services to the magazine. A reply arrived at once, inviting the young Dutchman, who had just completed his tour of duty, to see her in New York. Convinced that her correspondent was *the* Mrs. Kurt Weill, the editor rolled out the red carpet for Christiaan, securing for him audiences with Kenneth, Vidal Sassoon, and the Glemby Salon at Bergdorf Goodman.

Christiaan, however, chose to return to Holland to work with his father. From there he proceeded to Geneva in order to learn French while working as a UN barber. Finally, in 1967, curiosity drove him back to New York and the Bergdorf salon, where he was immediately appointed creative director. "Hair in America was still in the Lucy stage. You washed it, set it, teased it up to hide the roller marks, and coiffed the outer shell into a pleasing form." Christiaan, however, had brought with him from Holland the newest European hairdressers' implements — a roll brush and blow-dryer. With these tools he was able to eliminate the teasing phase of the wash-and-set, and produce softer 'dos that maintained their shape even when slept on. "It was sort of a transitional phase between stiff and more natural hair," he recalls.

"FORGIVEMETEAS"

"The timing was perfect. I was doing the right thing in the right place. Magazines began to take notice. It was also the moment when models switched from going to the salon for their hair to taking their stylist to the studio. This was the period of Twiggy, Penelope Tree, and Candice Bergen."

By 1969, Christiaan had had a dispute with the salon's management. "They wanted me to wear a blue suit — I preferred brown," he says. Christiaan had also helped pioneer the highly successful Bigi Cutaway, the younger, hipper division of Bergdorf's established salon, but he felt he had not been compensated in proportion to his contribution. "Anyway, magazines had been call-ing me so often, it made sense to leave." A full-fledged, full-time studio stylist, Christiaan soon fell into a long-term collaboration with Arthur Elgort, the master fashion photographer best known for his work for American *Vogue*. "Arthur has always been my favorite," he says without hesitation. "We are perfectly and mutu-ally compatible. We agree about how to get things done — which is basically never asking how to do it. We just come and do it. One of our biggest moments recently was getting white girls with dreadlocks into the front pages of *Vogue*," he says with obvious satisfaction. "What Arthur and I do I call 'out-of-life experiences.' It's what drives me — it's how I've found fun and joy with hair."

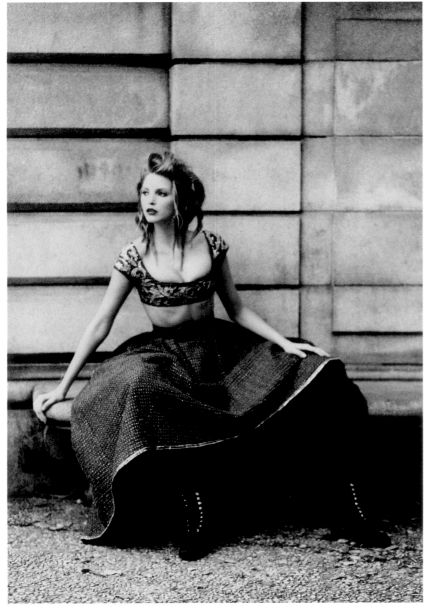

Nadja Auermann, photographed by Arthur Elgort for American *Vogue*.
Courtesy American *Vogue* ©The Condé Nast Publications Inc.

"DREADGRACE"

Nicole Kidman, photographed by Arthur Elgort for American *Vogue*.
Courtesy American *Vogue* ©The Condé Nast Publications Inc.

"HOLYMANE"

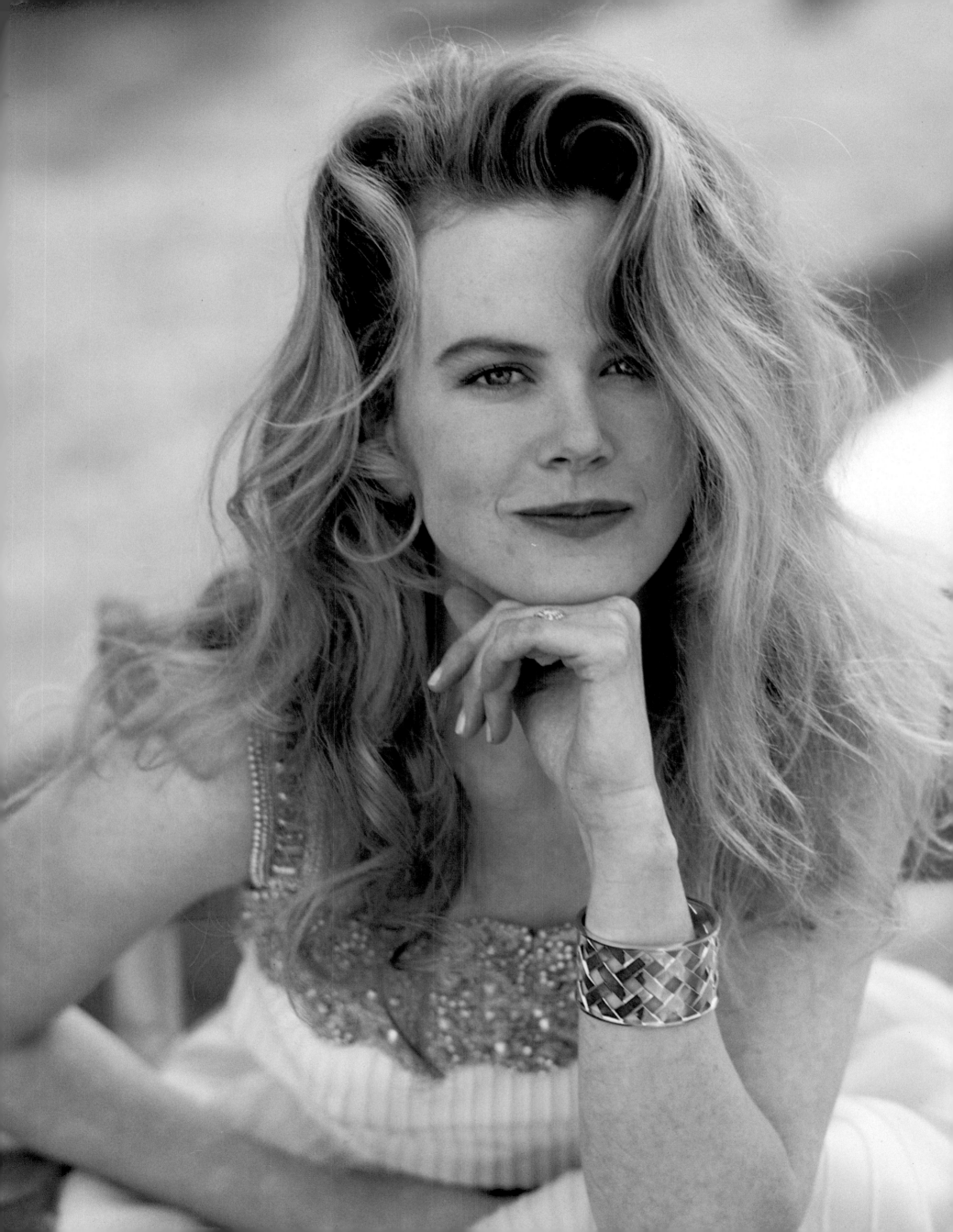

Likes

CUT:
self-cut

shaved heads

COLOR:
variety

grown-out roots

STYLE:
geometric shaping

satisfaction with hair from the inside out

TREATMENT:
rinsing with water instead of shampoo

Dislikes

CUT:
anything conventional

COLOR:
anything subtle

STYLE:
permed hair

worrying about the end result

extensions

bobby pins or any hairdo difficult to take down

insensitive touch

TREATMENT:
cleansing hair with commercial products

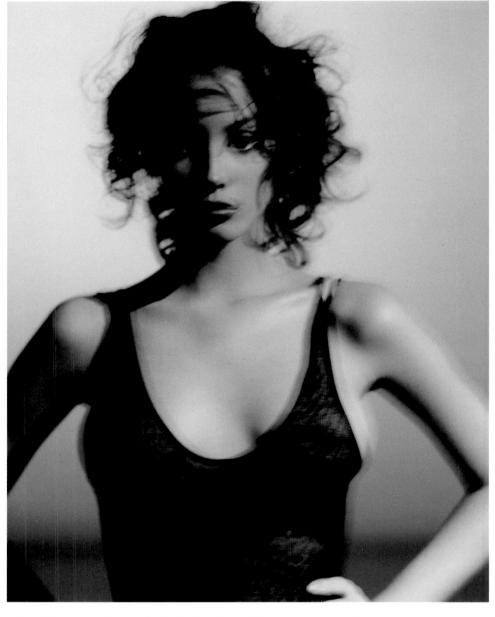

Christy Turlington, photographed by Arthur Elgort for *Interview*. Courtesy *Interview*

"WOCSYWAIF"

Cecilia Chancellor, photographed by Arthur Elgort for British *Vogue*. Courtesy British *Vogue* ©The Condé Nast Publications Ltd.

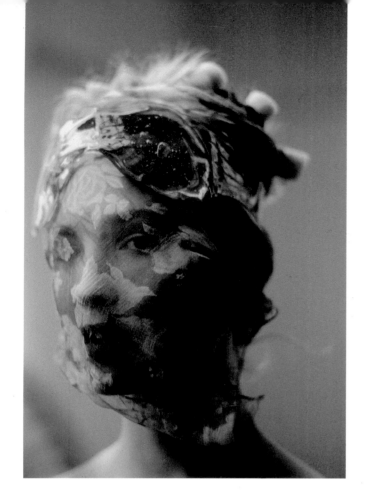

Photograph by Arthur Elgort for Italian *Vogue*. Courtesy Italian *Vogue*

"TWYLYTSTER"

Do's & Don'ts

Hair should mirror your mind, not your lover, your work, or your mother.

All hair has its own beauty.

In spite of stylists, hair in Western culture is still a pretty dull affair.

Love the hair you've got.

Hair is like a flower; it wakes up differently every day.

Clients

Grace Jones
Paloma Picasso
Debbie Harry
Nicole Kidman
Niki Taylor
Kate Moss
Christy Turlington
Stephen Sprouse

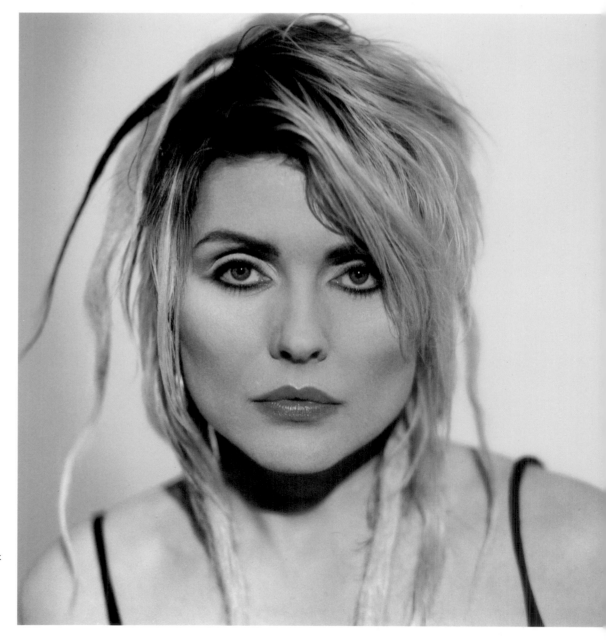

Debbie Harry, photographed by Arthur Elgort

"DEBHED"

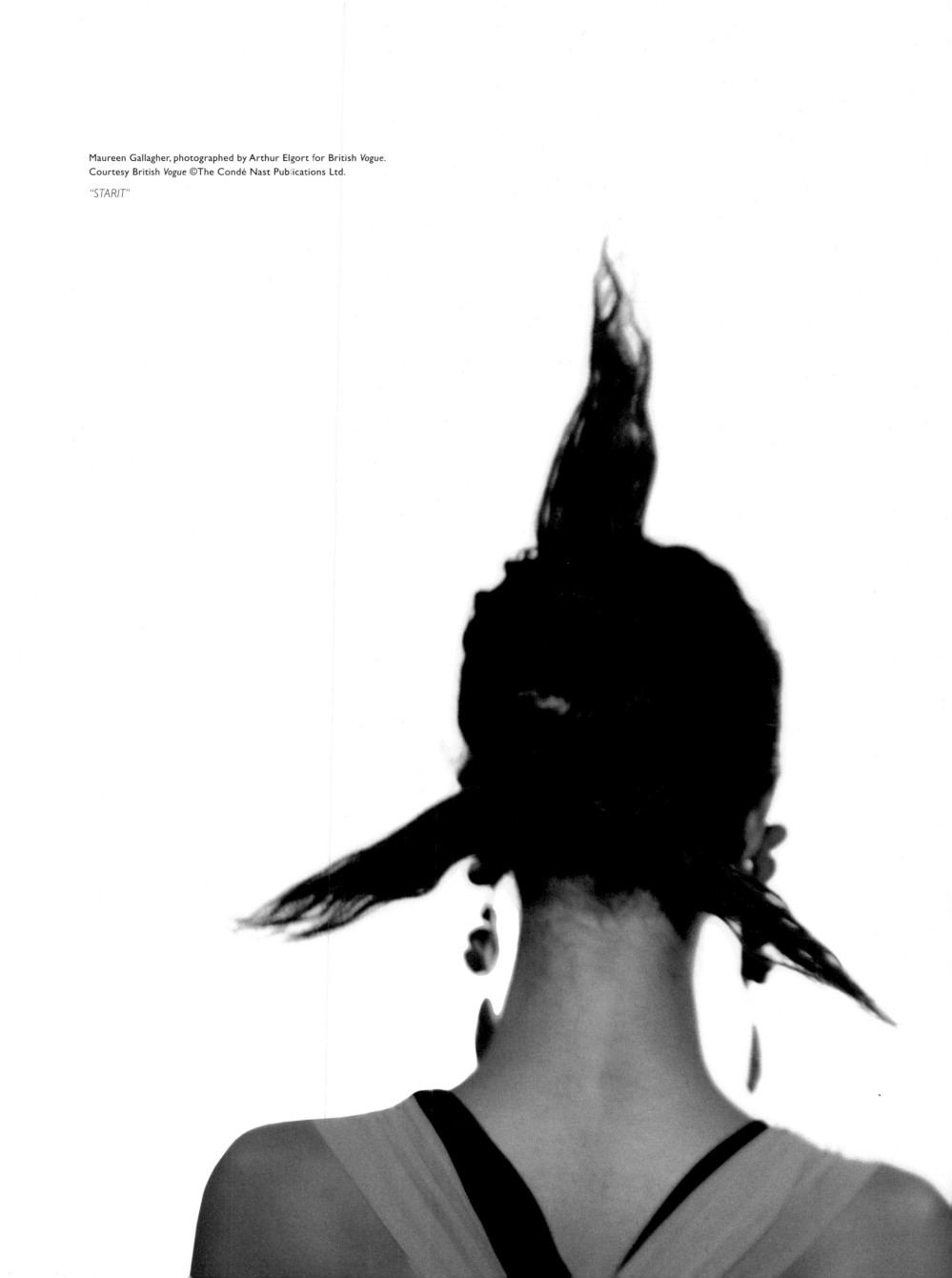

Maureen Gallagher, photographed by Arthur Elgort for British *Vogue*.
Courtesy British *Vogue* ©The Condé Nast Publications Ltd.

"STARIT"

Julien d'Ys

Ardent Artistry – Ancient Artifice

With his large, visionary eyes, spectral pallor, and waifishly delicate physique, Julien d'Ys has a distinctly other-worldly air – incongruous in a profession preoccupied with surfaces. He has a romantic's passion for history, particularly that of his native Brittany. It is not hard to imagine him as a displaced medieval spirit from that region, accidentally propelled into the glossy world he now inhabits. When speaking about his work, he is at a loss to explain his prodigious imagination. "When I arrive at a job, I never know what I'm going to do," he says in his quiet, ornately accented English. "It is a kind of magic that happens. I say to my angel, 'Help me! Help me!' I think it's something from God. It's very strange," he adds shyly. "If I'm asked to do something inspired by the 18th century, I suddenly feel as if I'm a hairdresser from that period."

D'Ys' guardian angel has apparently been nudging the stylist in the right direction, for some of model-dom's most memorable hair transformations have issued from his sorcerous scissors. Though many others claim credit, it was he who first clipped Linda Evangelista's long brunette tresses into a Beatles-style moptop in 1989, igniting a career that has burned brightly ever since. "The decision was made with Peter Lindbergh for an Italian *Vogue* shoot," d'Ys recalls. And it was his idea for Nadja Auermann to go platinum and wear her hair in a slight-ly cockeyed bob. "I wanted to make her look like Madeleine Soulogne, the French movie star of the 40s," he explains. No wonder he has won the affection of the single-name supermodels. "I don't like to torture the girls," he explains. "That's why they like me."

Ever since his childhood, women have been coaxing Julien to run his long, white fingers through their hair. When his grandmother broke her arm and was unable to put her hair up in her signature French twist, she called upon her young grandson to perform the duty. "She told me, 'Be a hairdresser. You'll always have money,'" he recalls. He practiced by "cutting my sister's hair and bleaching the hair of her Barbie doll." Within the family

Linda Evangelista, photographed by Peter Lindbergh for Italian *Vogue*. Courtesy Italian *Vogue*

"I wanted to evoke a modern Ava Gardner, with a touch of Argentine tango."

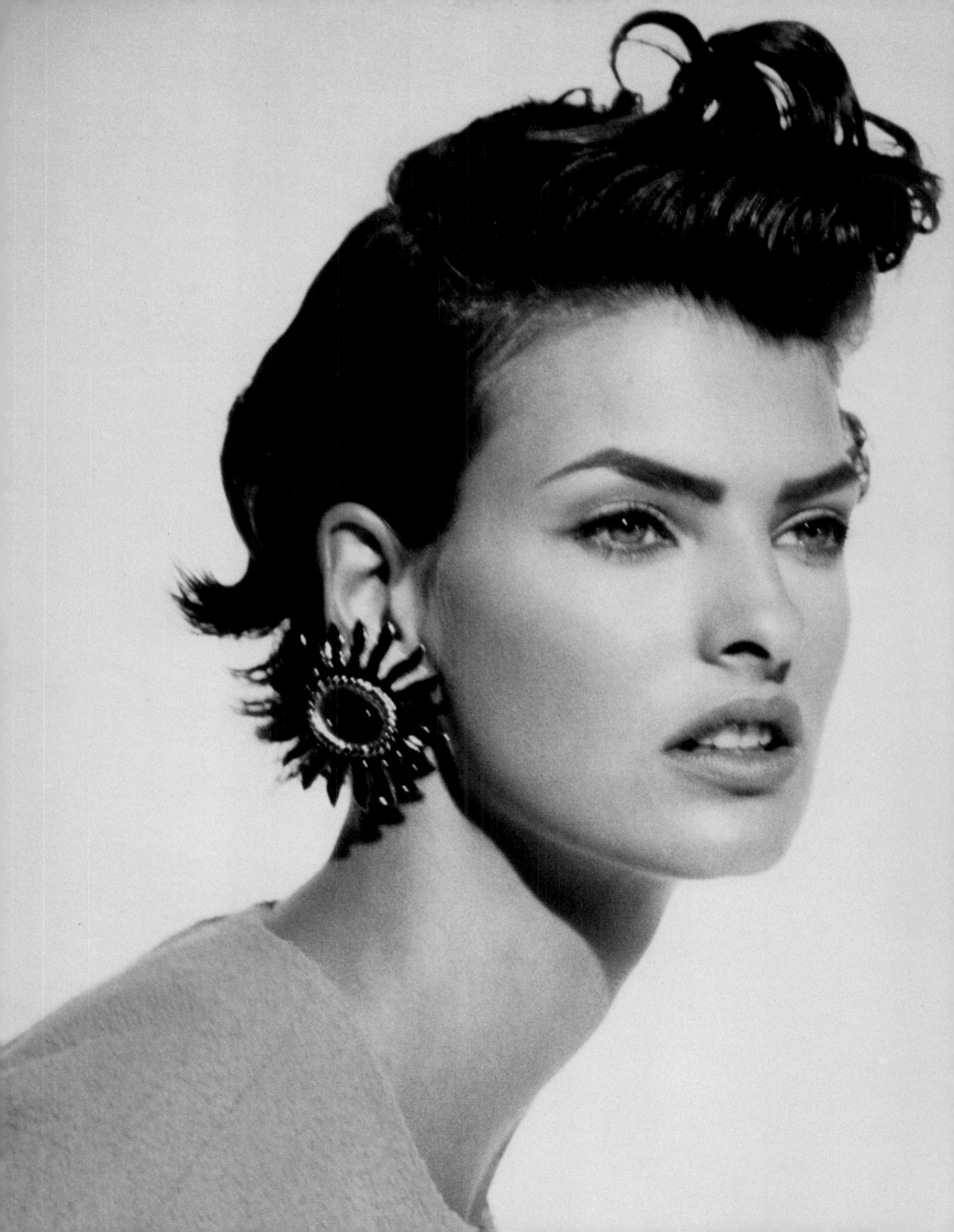

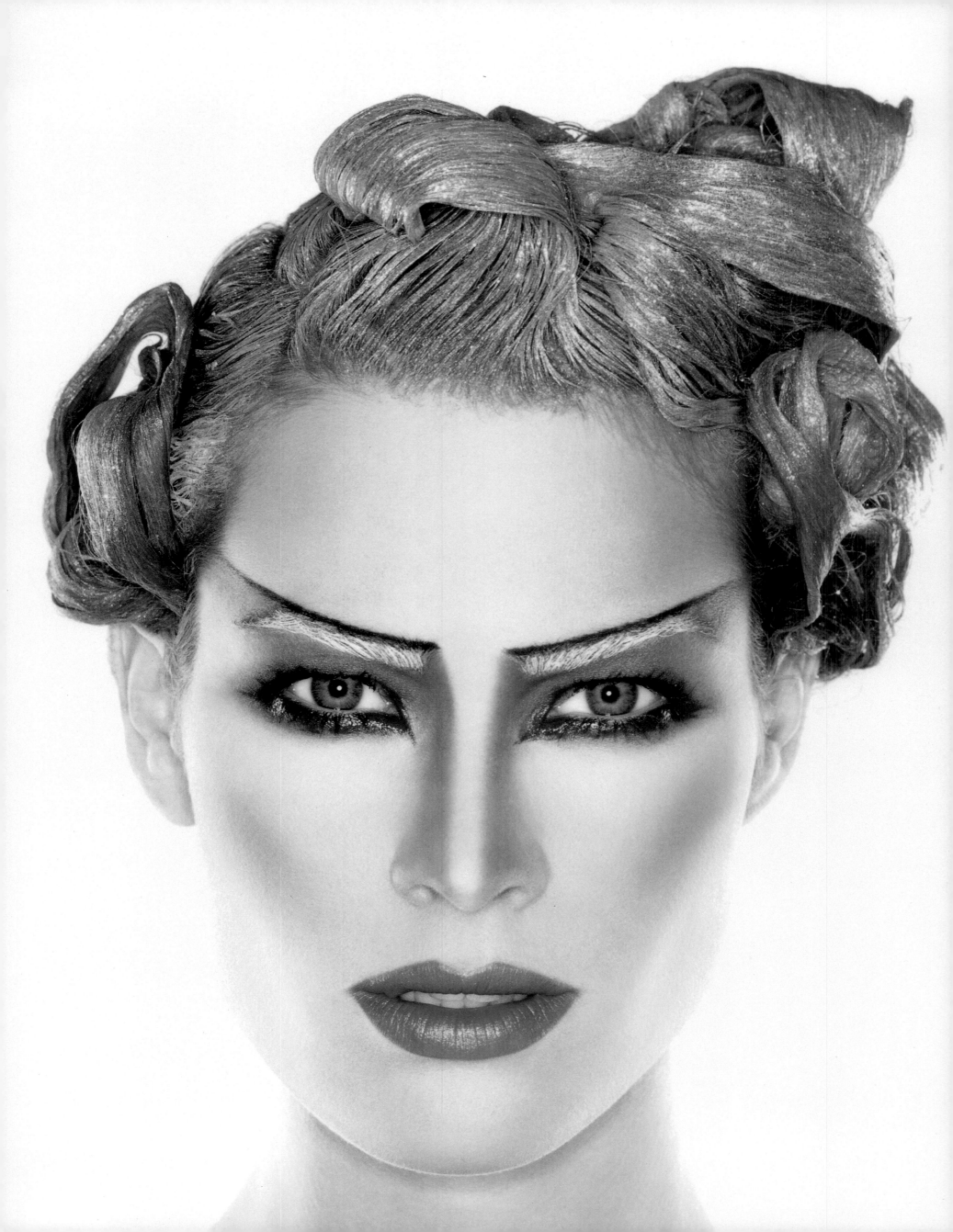

circle, his mother, too, was "a big influence. She's brilliant. She always had her long hair cut short like a boy, even in the 50s. She looked like Bettina," the legendary Parisian model and mistress of Aly Khan.

D'Ys' early fascination with hair was complemented by a passion for painting and sculpture, two avocations he still pursues assiduously. "I wanted to attend the Ecole des Beaux-Arts in Paris, but my father was opposed," he says. Instead, d'Ys attended architecture school and studied interior decoration, but after two years he dropped out. "I hate learning things from school," he says. At age 18 he completed a one-year tour of duty with the French Marines, serving his country "by cutting the hair of all the men on the boat." Though constrained to give only regulation haircuts, he still managed to be "very creative with scissors." Next he took a job at a small salon in the village of Verrière-le-Buisson, one hour from Paris, where he shampooed the hair of two of France's most illustrious *littéraires*: the statesman and novelist André Malraux and the aristocratic Louise de Vilmorin, author of *Madame de, . . .* "They both had big heads, they were so intelligent," d'Ys recalls. "But I learned from my mother never to be impressed, never to ask for autographs. That was the very

beginning of my career with hair. I was very worried. I thought my voice would change and become like a lady's!"

If his vocal pitch did not rise, the degree of his professionalism did. When one of the girls at the village salon left for Paris to work at the famous Jean Louis David salon, d'Ys, intrigued, "followed her there. I saw the director of the salon, who asked me to do an essay, which I performed on the girlfriend of my sister. Three hours later I was hired," he reports, still pleased at the memory. Soon he began "working like crazy, crazy – weekends and nights – doing hair for *Marie Claire*, and French *Vogue*," with such photographers as Hans Feurer, Paolo Roversi, and Peter Lindbergh. The hot young stylist, who looked all of 15, then jumped to the Daniel Harlow salon, "a trendy 80s spot," where he cut Ines de la Fressange's hair and continued with his studio work. "I've always loved working with a team," he says ardently. "I like the creativity of collaborating. I am unhappy to see people in the fashion profession becoming more and more businesslike."

D'Ys made the inevitable move to New York, where, to his delight, he found himself working with such legends as Andy Warhol (for a *Vogue Bambini* shoot), Robert Mapplethorpe, Horst,

Facing page and right: **Meghan Douglas**, photographed by Michael Thompson for W. Courtesy W

"This was a Barbarella/Superwoman comic book look. I teased it up very big and messy, with lots of hairspray. I like the short fringe on her face."

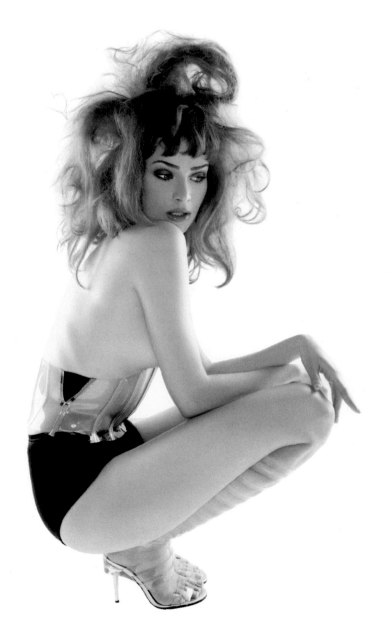

"Stephane Marais, the makeup artist, and I attempted something almost Cubist, very planar, like the paintings of Tamara de Lempicka. I wanted the hair to be curled, almost like wood shavings. First I sculpted her hair with clay, rather like an algae mask for the face, then sprayed it with colored hairspray and touches of glitter hairspray."

Hairstory

STYLIST: *Julien d'Ys*
SALON ADDRESS: *None*
PLACE OF BIRTH: *Douarnenez, France*
FIRST JOB: *Age 20, National Service in the French Navy*
TRADEMARKS: *Good teamwork; Fervor for fantasy and historical periods; Radical approach to hair; Comforting clients*

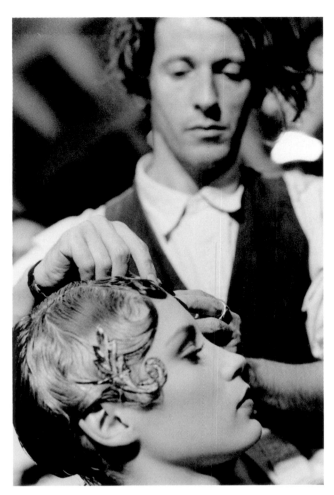

Julien d'Ys with Olga, photographed by Juliette Butler for Chanel Couture

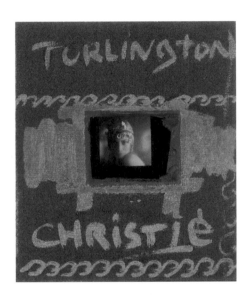

Christy Turlington, photographed by Julien d'Ys for Chanel Couture

"For each show I keep a little scrapbook. I gave it a touch of gold because the theme for the show was gold."

Avedon, and Geoffrey Beene. He also fondly remembers styling hair for a 1986 Stephen Sprouse show (in conjunction with his colleague Christiaan). "I made the hair completely flat, at a time when everyone else was doing big hair," he says proudly. But unlike most of his expatriate confreres' relocations, d'Ys' transplant to New York did not take. "The mid-80s were a crazy time, between the coke and AIDS. That's why I returned to France. I love my country. New York is so inspiring, but it drives you mad if you stay too long." His Paris home base, he feels, keeps him at a sanity-preserving remove from the New York fashion mafia. Far from being the stereotypical temperamental diva, he likes riding the subway, socializing with obscure artists, and going fly-fishing for recreation. "This business already takes enough out of my life," he explains. Nevertheless, he wouldn't object to finding an atelier in New York where he could concentrate on making his clay sculptures and oil paintings, colorful figurative works executed on paper.

Paris by itself provides enough stimulation — even from within the many ranks of fashion. "I've learned a lot from Karl Lagerfeld," he says. "With him I've worked on the image for Chloé, Karl Lagerfeld, and Chanel. Karl told me that he wants me to do some hair for Chanel — long, all the way to the floor. I have

to find some wigs! Fashion goes so fast these days. I think it's Karl who has accelerated the pace. I can keep up, but it makes many people go nuts."

Though d'Ys claims that in his work he thinks only of the future. "Even to do this book, I found it hard to look back." Despite this, he has a nostalgic reverence for many of the hair-care traditions of the past. "I try to find new ideas in old ones," he says. Many of these recommendations come straight out of the kitchen cupboard. He suggests, for example, a potion of vodka and lemon for bleaching hair, and a combination of sugar and water as a substitute for hairspray or setting lotion. "Chemically, I don't think there's that much difference. In the 40s, a lot of women used sugar and water as a fixative. And it always interested me that in Brittany old women put butter on their hair as a kind of gel." One of d'Ys' aunts, a beautiful woman who sang opera, has also been "an important inspiration to me. She had hair down to her knees. To wash it she would put it in long braids, and apply to them a mixture of rum and eggs. Most people get disgusted when I tell them that story! But we shouldn't be limited by our familiar routines and daily habits. When I go into the studio, it's as if it's my first time working. For me it's always new."

Nadja Auermann, photographed by Karl Lagerfeld for Chanel Couture

"Here I used a large pearl ornament, almost like a hatpin, in homage to Chanel, who loved pearls. This style was inspired by antiquity, by a Greek statue."

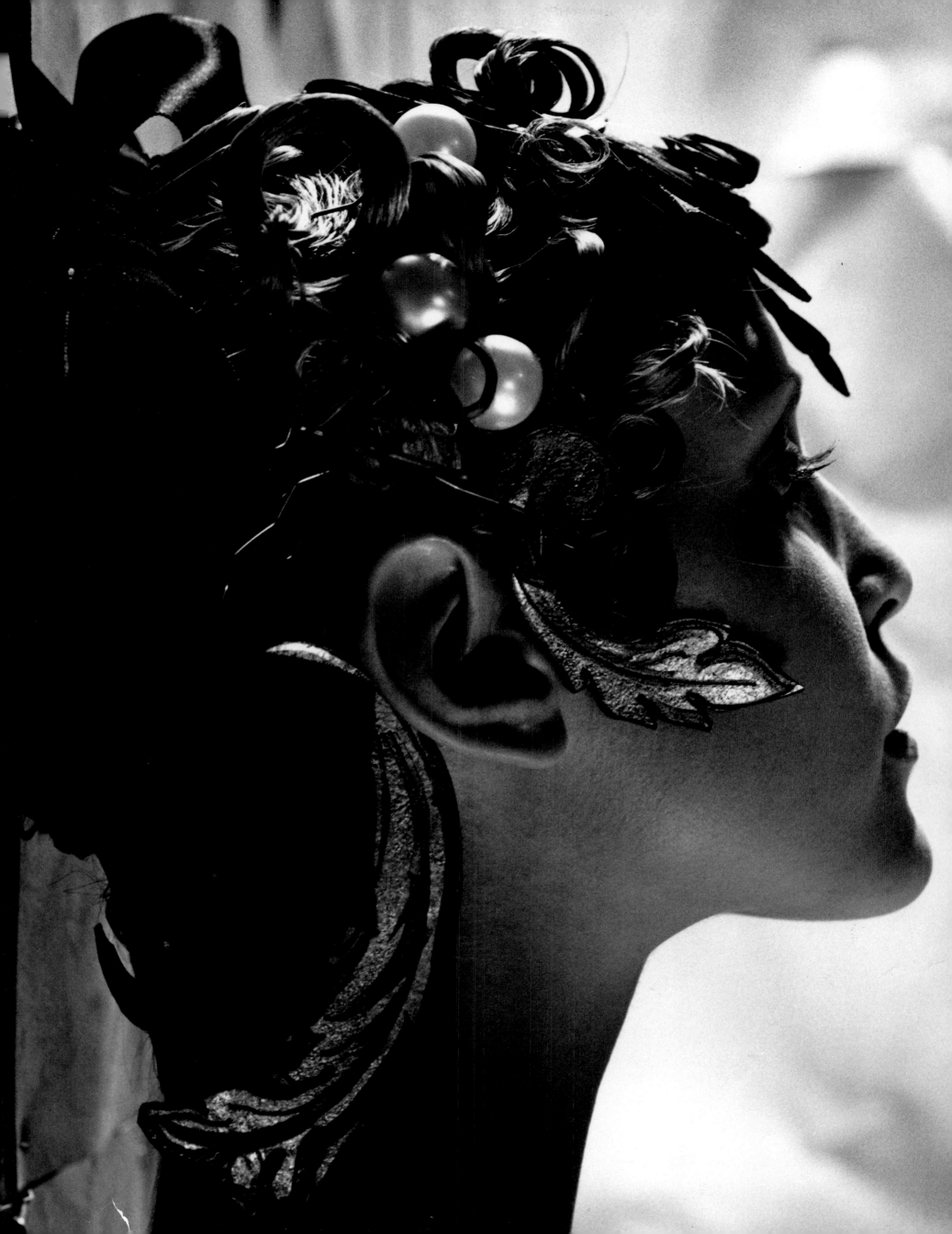

Do's & Don'ts

I think women looked amazing in the 1940s and 50s. People live too quickly today. Their busy lives don't allow for them to take pleasure in their toilette, to do something special for a party. I'm all for bringing back the idea of women taking time to consider their looks. When women spent more time in the salon, it was a pampered time for them, not just slavish ritual. It involved taking time out, and the benefit, beyond the beauty aspect, was relaxation – time for themselves, almost like Zen or yoga.

The upcoming looks will be pulled together, but keeping the hair flat on top is one way to keep it modern. To add volume in the back (that "poof" that is showing up on all the fashion pages), roll the back section in two or three large rollers. Back comb or tease it for volume, then smooth over the top and spray it.

I hate vulgarity. Some of the looks shown here may seem very extreme, but each has its own elegance.

For a woman with a heavy neck, it often works well to have hair that moves upward, away from the face, to bring the focus higher and make a statement, a statement about softness.

After the hair is washed, I like to rinse it in a bit of vinegar. This is an old trick that makes it very shiny.

As women get older, some try to hide behind their hair, to cover their face with too much hair. I prefer to see the hair pulled back, or cropped short. Both are styles that suit a woman's age, but are more modern. My mama is from Brittany, and although she is quite stocky now, she was thin in her youth and always preferred wearing short, men's hairstyles, which she had cut at a barber shop. Now, when I cut her hair, she still likes it very short. It makes her feel very light and free. When it is longer, she feels heavy. My sister, however, has long hair that cascades down her back. That's the style she likes, and I would never cut it. Every woman is different, of course, and it is impossible to generalize.

Nadja Auermann, photographed by Karl Lagerfeld for Chanel Couture

"The hair was curled flat, sprayed, and then adorned with Chanel accessories."

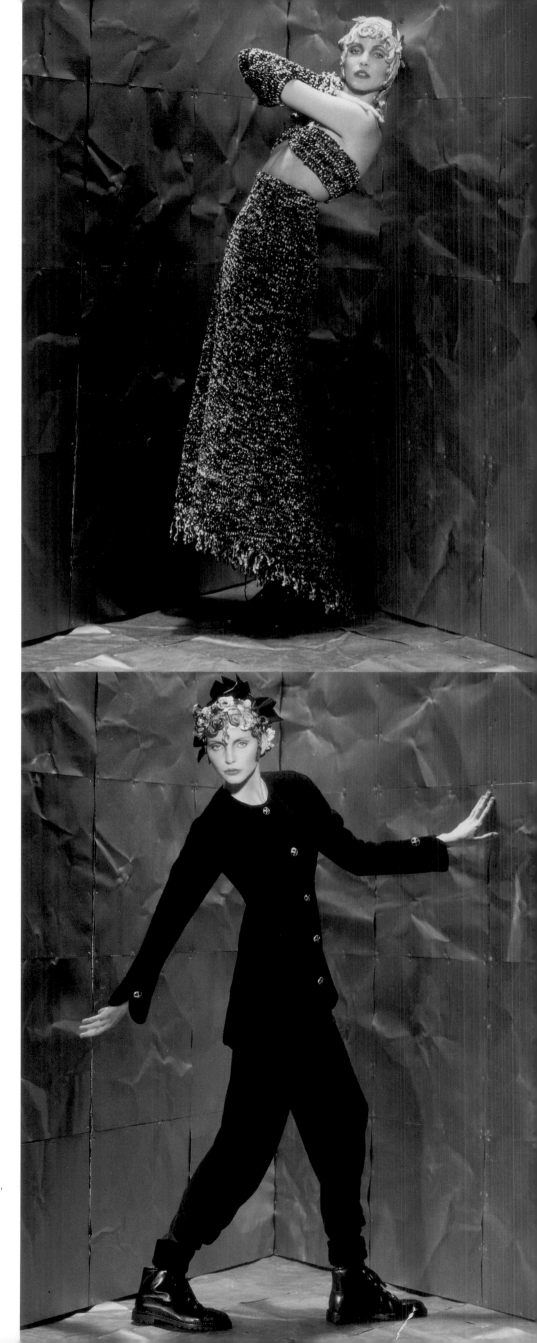

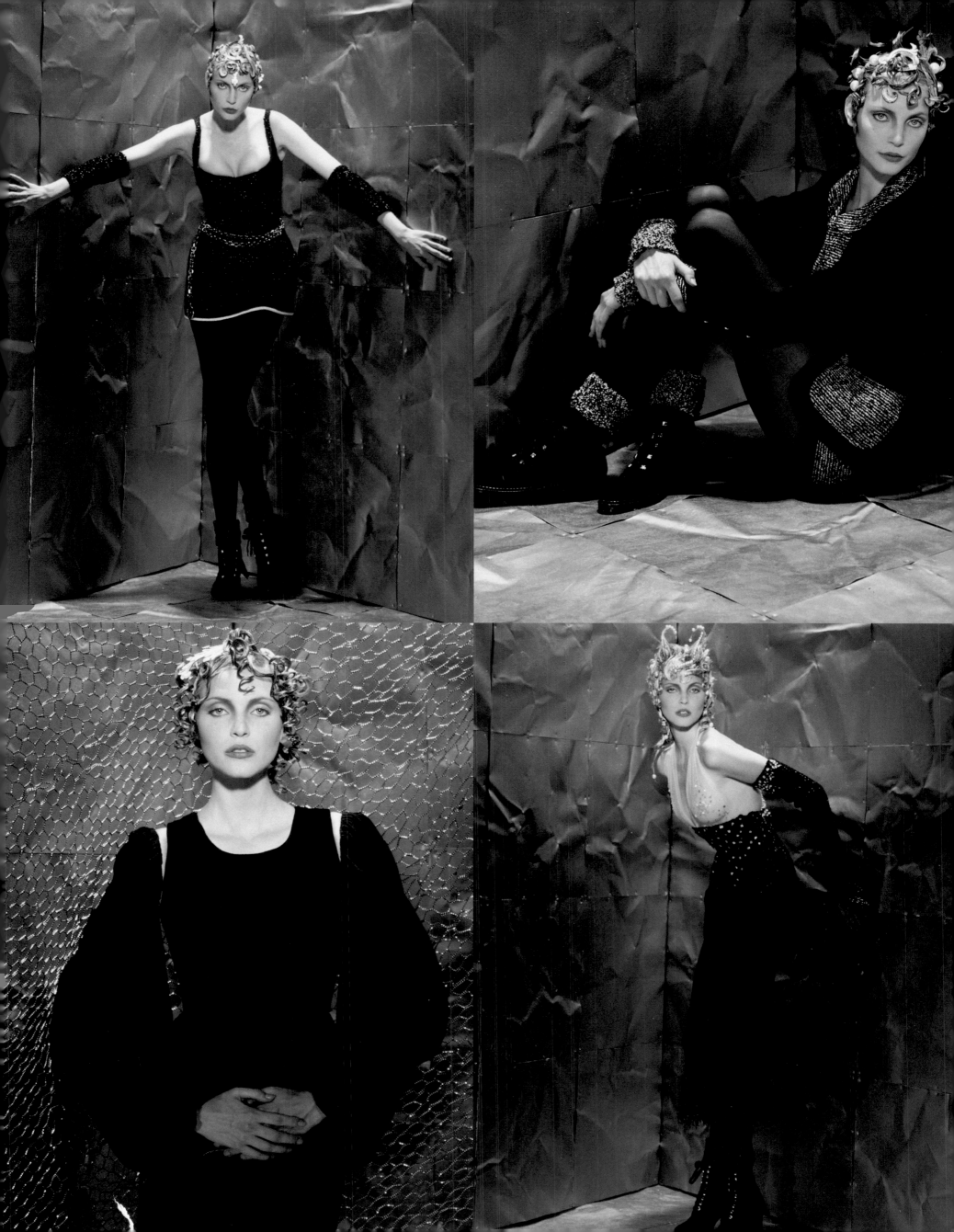

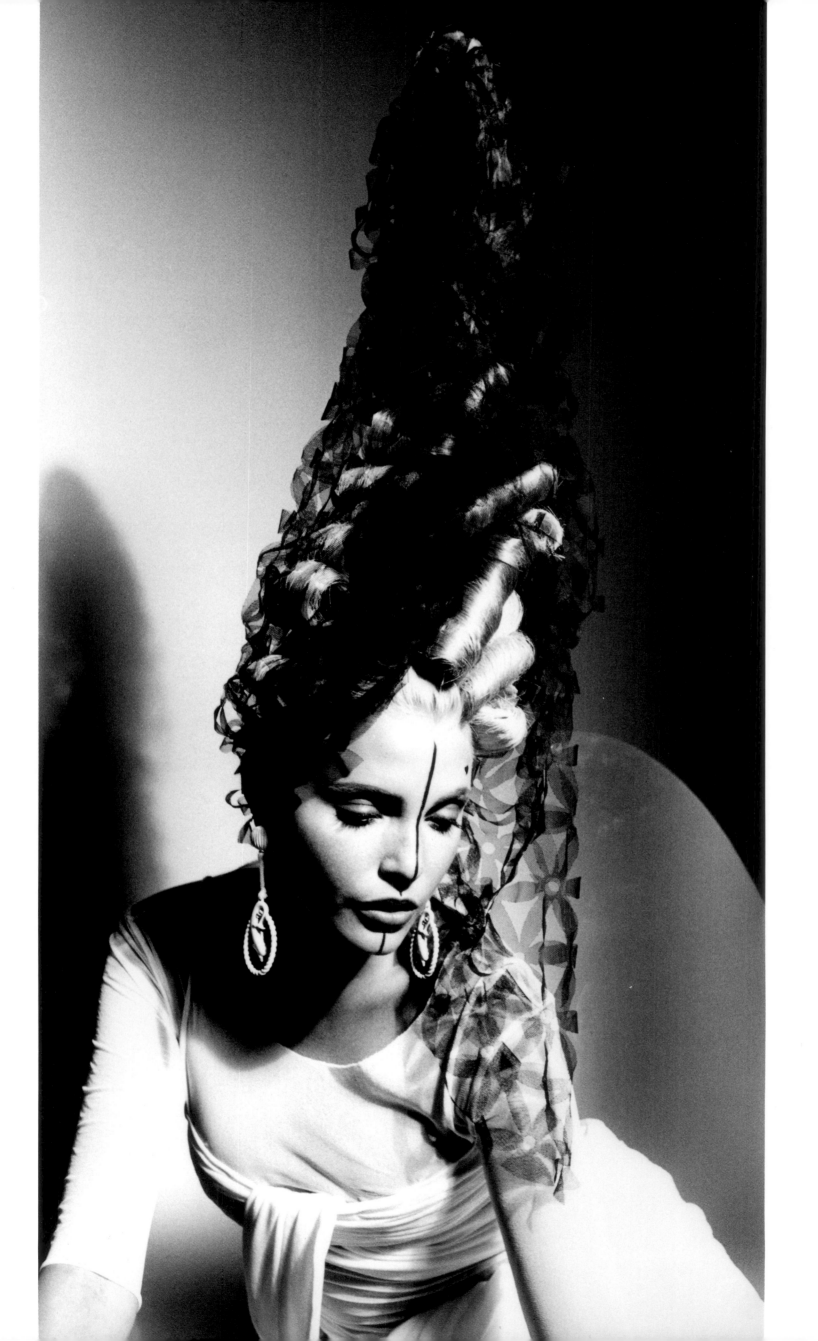

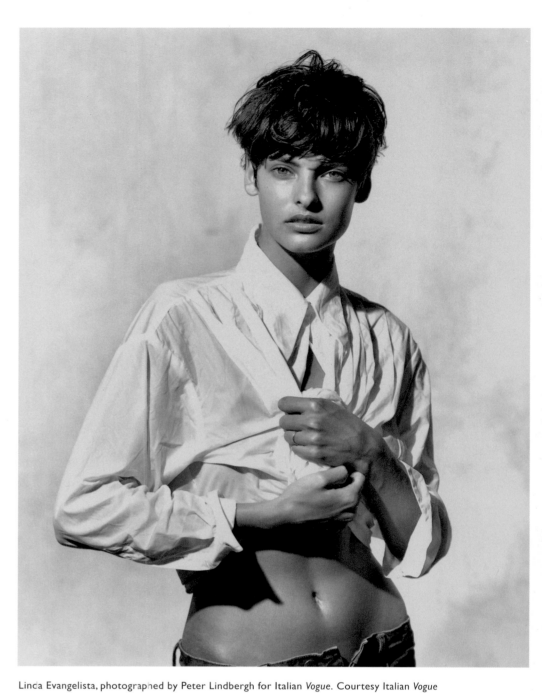

Linda Evangelista, photographed by Peter Lindbergh for Italian *Vogue*. Courtesy Italian *Vogue*

"This haircut re-launched the bob in 1989. She went from very long to short – inspired by the little boy's cut of the Beatles."

Nadja Auermann, photographed by Karl Lagerfeld for Karl Lagerfeld

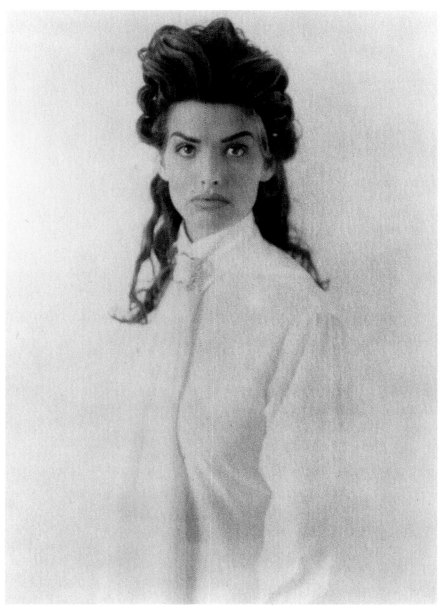

Shana, photographed by Paolo Roversi for French *Vogue*. Courtesy French *Vogue*

"All the hair is back in a tight chignon. The hairpiece was painted with acrylic to give it form; it felt like rubber. The idea here was to do a contemporary version of an elaborate Japanese Kabuki high chignon."

Likes

CUT:
boyishly short or extremely long

COLOR:
either subtle and natural, or glamorously extreme

STYLE:
wigs
hair extensions
braids
playfulness with hair and with life
combination of a little messiness and a lot of imagination
hair creations with cultural and historical references

TREATMENT:
old-fashioned home concoctions
vodka and lemon to lighten hair
rum and egg mixture to wash hair

Dislikes

STYLE:
perms or bleached hair
not questioning and updating your hair habits

Kim Williams, photographed by Peter Lindbergh for *Gilles*

"For an Egyptian style, like that of Nefertiti, I used Afro hairpieces in different colors, all blowing in the wind."

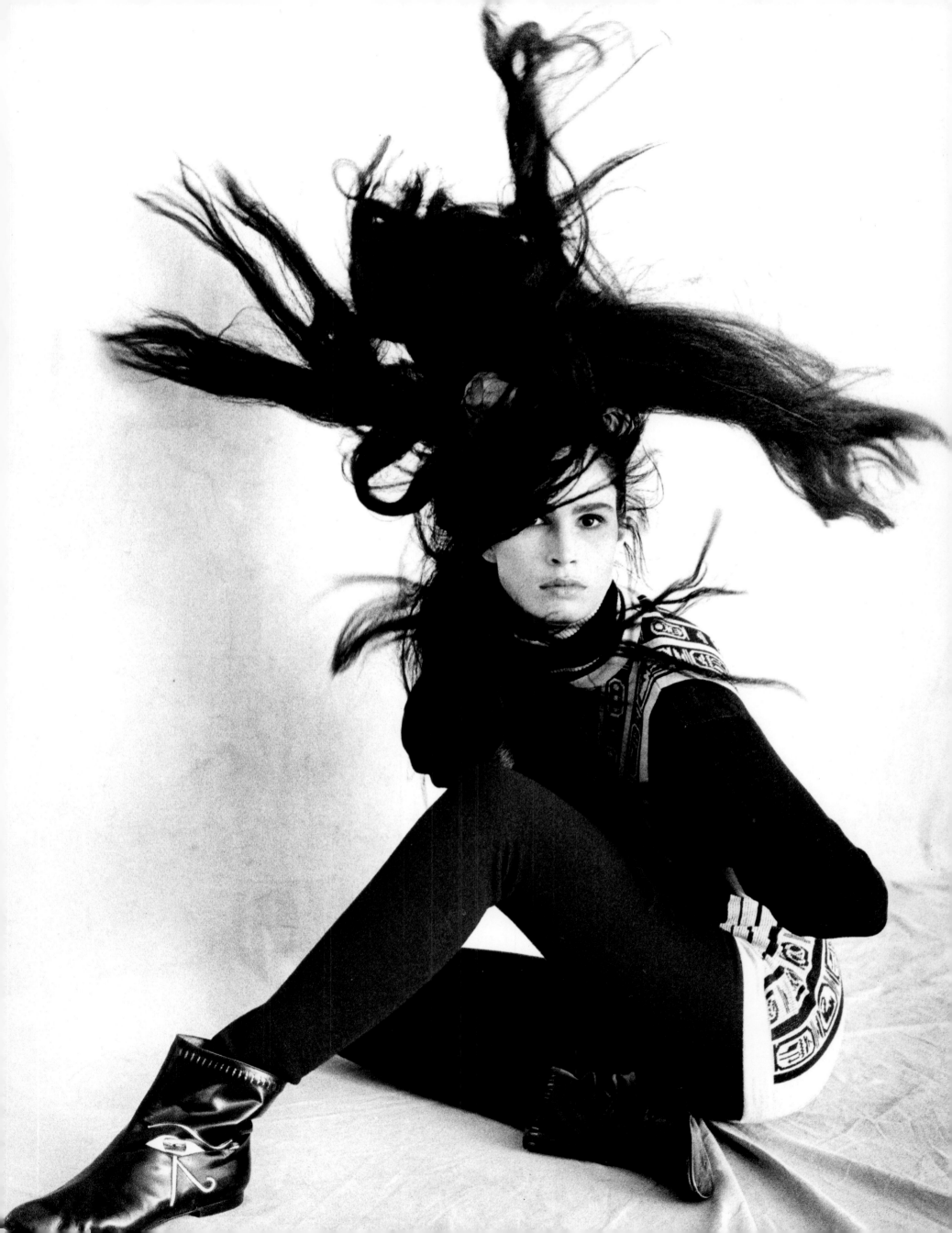

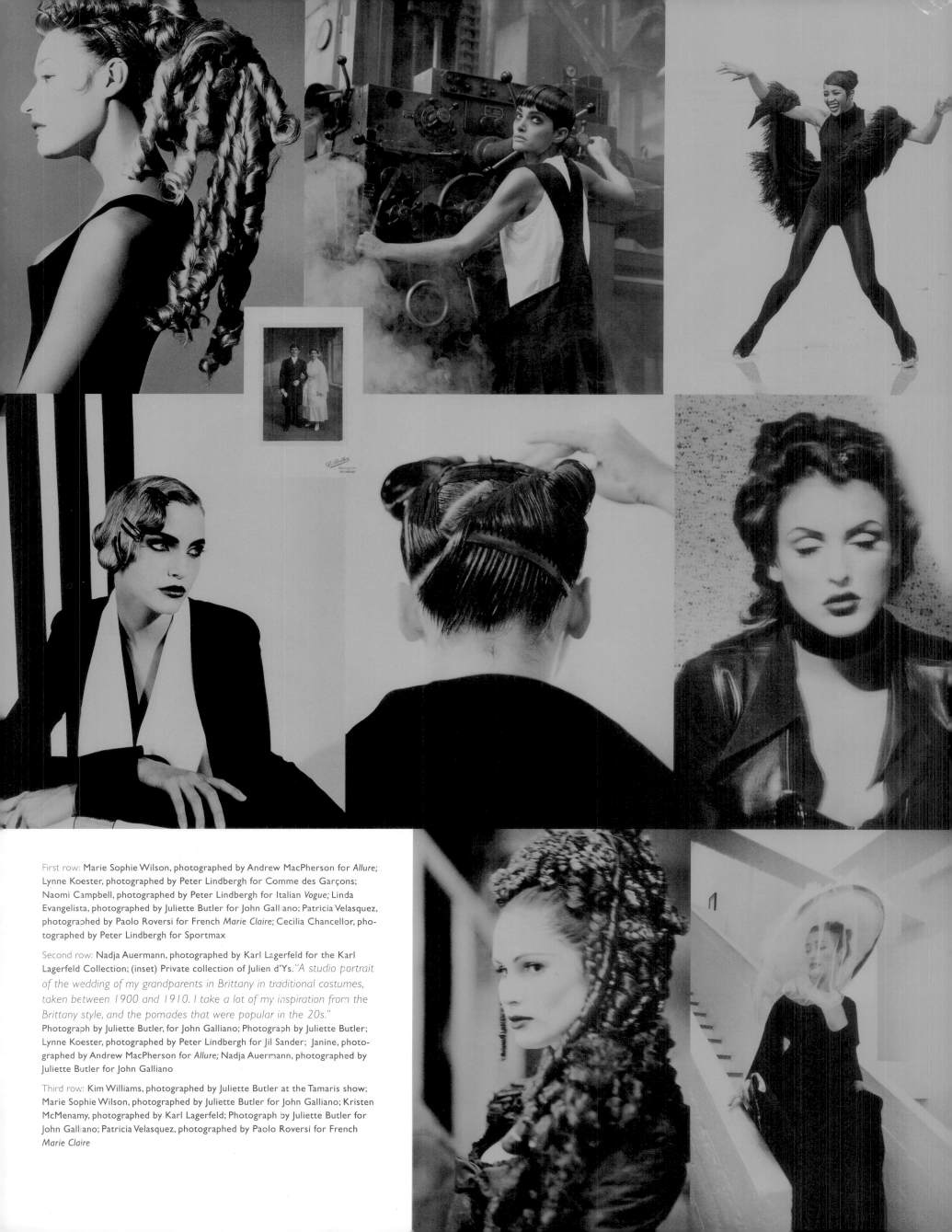

First row: Marie Sophie Wilson, photographed by Andrew MacPherson for *Allure*; Lynne Koester, photographed by Peter Lindbergh for Comme des Garçons; Naomi Campbell, photographed by Peter Lindbergh for Italian *Vogue*; Linda Evangelista, photographed by Juliette Butler for John Galliano; Patricia Velasquez, photographed by Paolo Roversi for French *Marie Claire*; Cecilia Chancellor, photographed by Peter Lindbergh for Sportmax

Second row: Nadja Auermann, photographed by Karl Lagerfeld for the Karl Lagerfeld Collection; (inset) Private collection of Julien d'Ys. *"A studio portrait of the wedding of my grandparents in Brittany in traditional costumes, taken between 1900 and 1910. I take a lot of my inspiration from the Brittany style, and the pomades that were popular in the 20s."* Photograph by Juliette Butler, for John Galliano; Photograph by Juliette Butler; Lynne Koester, photographed by Peter Lindbergh for Jil Sander; Janine, photographed by Andrew MacPherson for *Allure*; Nadja Auermann, photographed by Juliette Butler for John Galliano

Third row: Kim Williams, photographed by Juliette Butler at the Tamaris show; Marie Sophie Wilson, photographed by Juliette Butler for John Galliano; Kristen McMenamy, photographed by Karl Lagerfeld; Photograph by Juliette Butler for John Galliano; Patricia Velasquez, photographed by Paolo Roversi for French *Marie Claire*

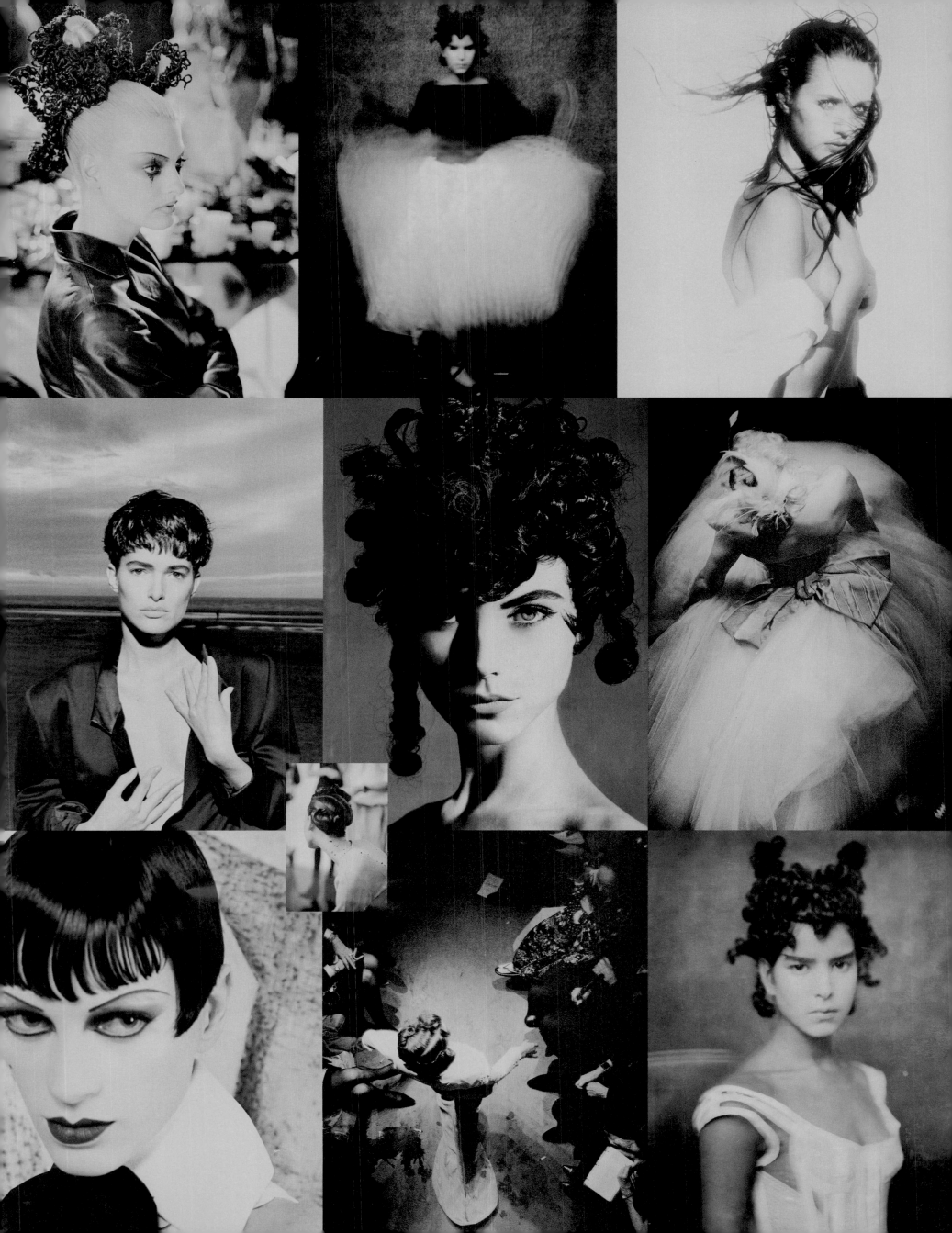

Clients

Andy Warhol

Robert Mapplethorpe

Catherine Deneuve

Isabella Rossellini

Madonna

Isabelle Adjani

Nadja Auermann

Linda Evangelista

Karl Lagerfeld

Comme des Garçons

Lindsay, photographed by Peter Lindbergh for Comme des Garçons

"The Angel. Lindsay has such a young, almost saint-like look. I clipped her hair back so it appears to be short, but you can still see some different lengths. Then it was shaped with gel.'

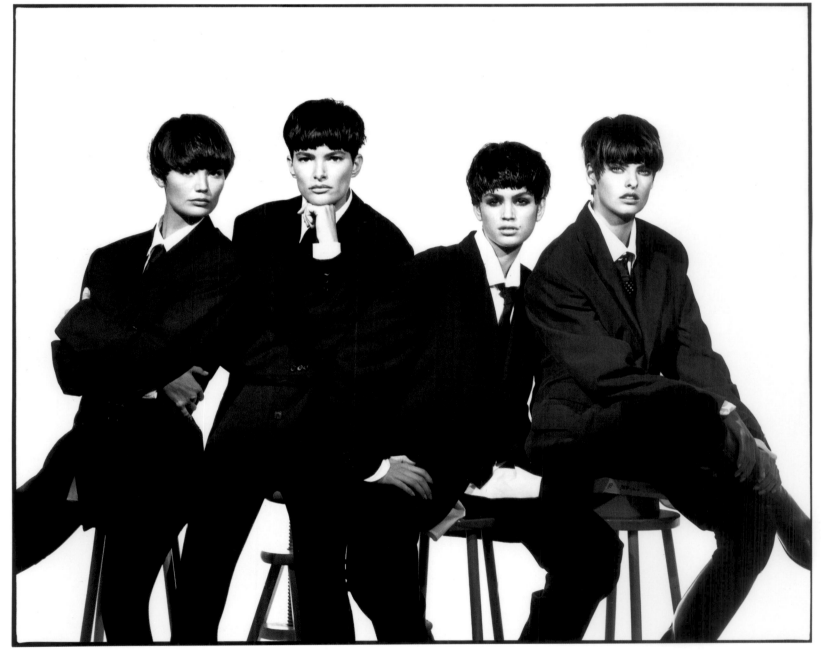

Uli, Lynne Koester, Cindy Crawford, and Linda Evangelista, photographed by Peter Lindbergh for Italian *Vogue*. Courtesy Italian *Vogue*

"The 'Fab Four' Beatles look. The only one wearing a wig is Cindy Crawford."

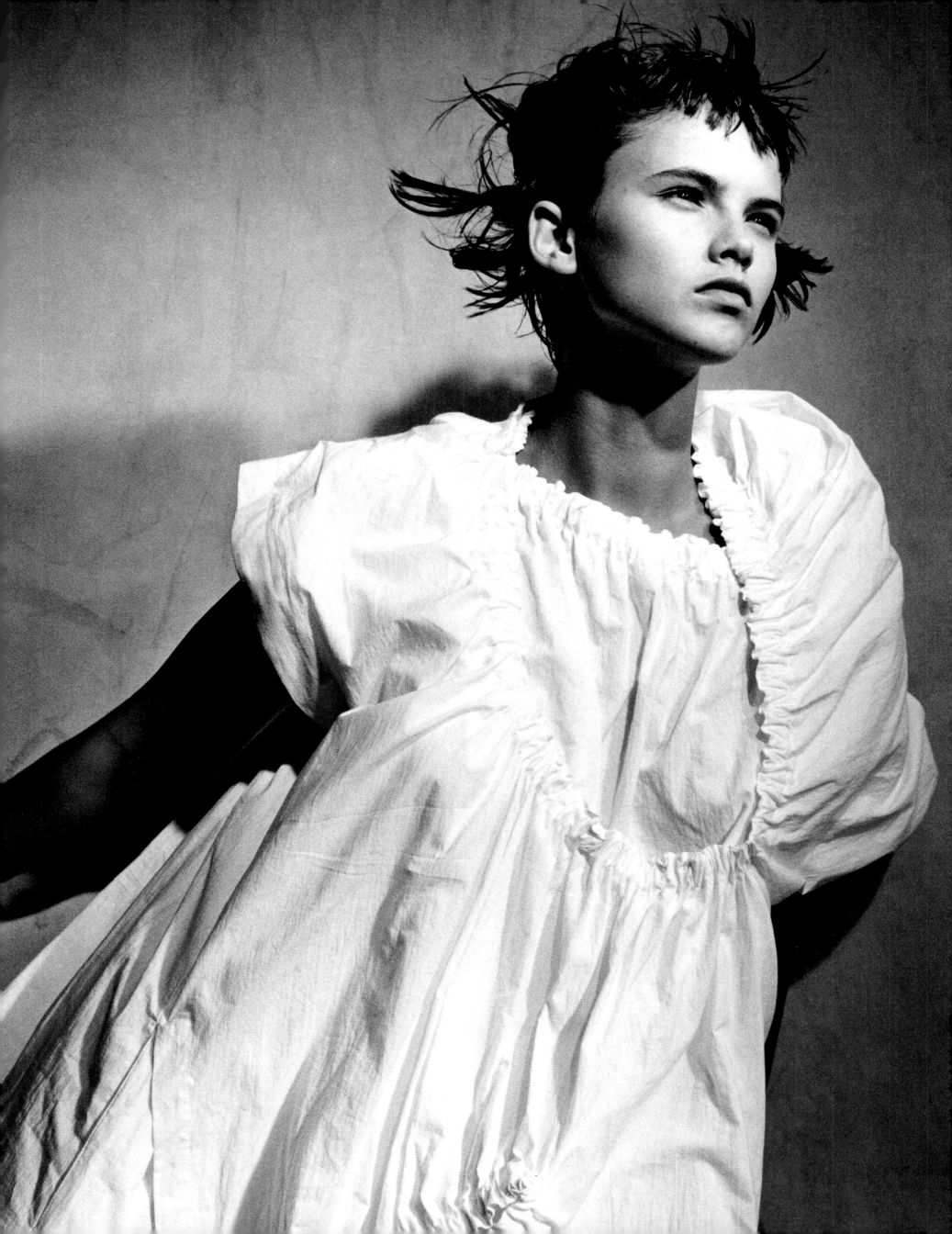

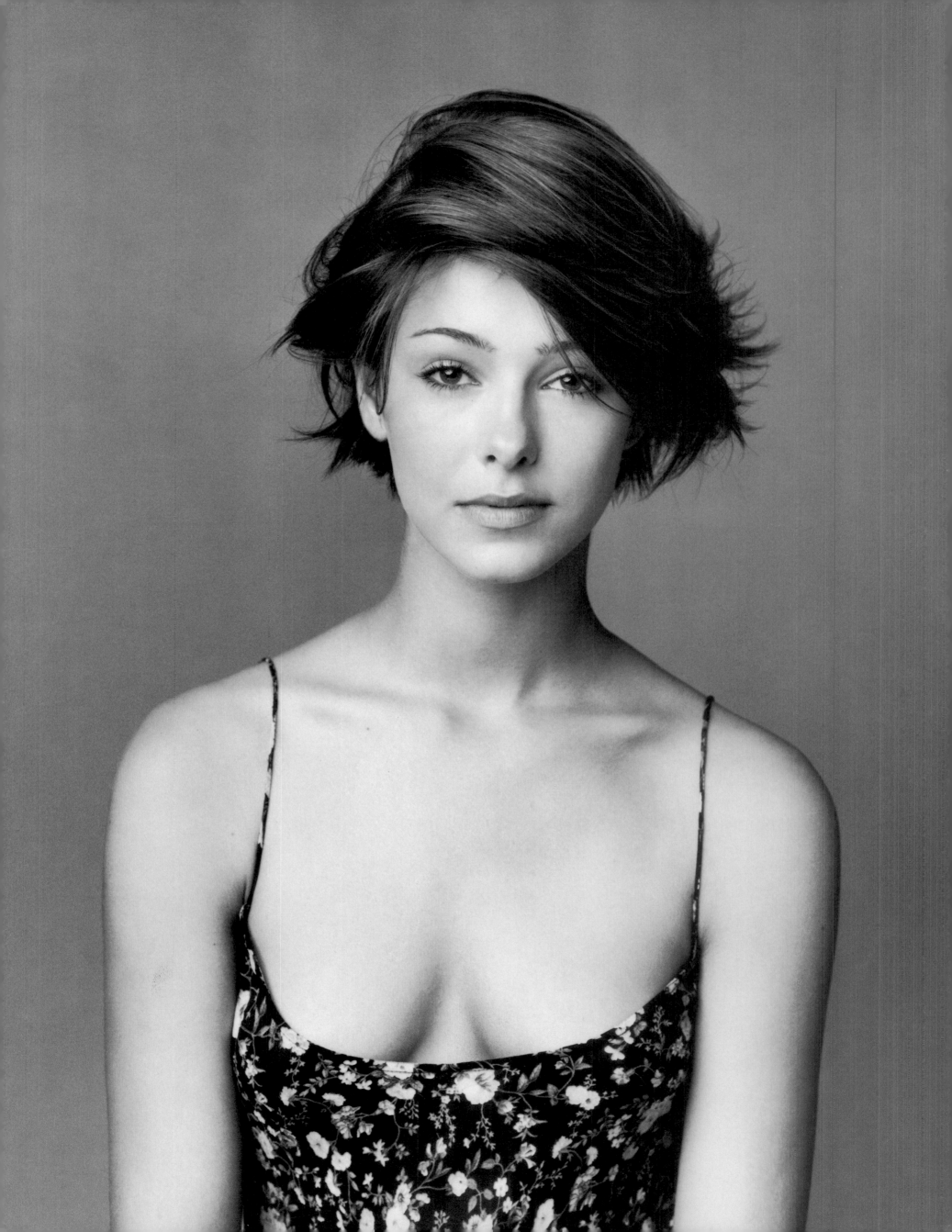

FREDERIC FEKKAI

Deep Cuts

Entering the vast Frederic Fekkai Beauty Center, situated on Bergdorf Goodman's seventh floor, is like plunging into the heart of a luxurious beehive. Phalanxes of uniformed staff, many of whom are refugees from obscure salons, welcome the visitor with honeyed greetings. "How may I help you, love?" one male receptionist inquires solicitously. There are the myriad curving cells, one neatly abutting the next, where cutting, drying, consultations, manicures, coloring, and confessions take place. There is the perpetual, purposeful darting, from station to station and from client to client, of worker bees and queen bees — assistants and stylists — all on the brink of collision as they serve tea, carry coats, brush bits of hair from patrons' shoulders, transmit messages. As background to all this movement, there is the incessant hum of countless blow-dryers — deafening at first, but soon receding into a kind of aural-wallpaper white noise.

From behind a chair in this nest of hyperactivity emerges a singular figure — a raven-haired, sloe-eyed man with smiling cupid's-bow lips and wearing an immaculate white shirt monogrammed with the "ff" logo. This is the eponymous, $290-a-head Frederic Fekkai, and he has just finished clipping the hair of a strapping fellow, who is left to admire his carefully shorn image in the mirror opposite him. Fekkai, his hovering assistant Tricia warns, is already an hour and a half behind schedule and must proceed without delay to his next client. It is already 4:30 and he has at least a dozen more cuts to perform before closing time. Fekkai, in contrast to Tricia, is all calm, easy charm.

[4:30 PM] Fekkai arrives at another station, where a wet-haired, middle-aged woman patiently awaits him. She is grateful, not at all reproachful, as he runs his smooth fingers through her sparse hair. "Each time I change the haircut," Fekkai explains, his words keeping tempo with his rapid snipping, "I never want to copy what I've done before. I keep the same spirit, but I make a different style." He maneuvers with such speed, and applies such mental concentration, that just to observe him is exhausting. "I don't get tired," he says, zestfully. "Only a little bit here in my shoulders and neck, after a long day. A massage will take care of that. And why wouldn't I work quickly? I know exactly what I'm doing." The client, petite and bony, offers her testimonial. "I've been seeing

Frederic for three and a half years. I've been to them all. Frederic is the best in the world. He's a genius." And how did she arrive at that judgment? "He does what's best for your kind of hair," she says with the immutable conviction of a true believer. "I have extremely thin hair. He makes it look thicker." Fekkai explains that he achieves fullness through "a distribution of layers over a one-length base." The face-framing layers soften the features, accentuate the cheekbones, and "respect the hairline." Each layer melds into the next, permitting the hair to move fluidly rather than choppily. Shaping "goes with the flow of the bone structure, the profile, and the proportions of the body" – which is why he asks every client to stand for part of the cutting session. "I want to do wash-and-wear hair. It has to work even if it's stormy or raining. And she can style the cut to be either sophisticated or casual." The client corrects her hairdresser. "There *is* no styling," she asserts emphatically. "Frederic's haircuts style themselves." The blow-dry, as always, is left to an assistant – Fekkai's over-booked schedule doesn't allow for such lingering attentions – but he will be back to inspect the results. Amazingly enough, once dried, the woman's cunningly clipped, baby-fine wisps fluff up into a sexy, look-making mane.

[4:45 PM] Fekkai hastens over to the next patron. Like a doctor making his bedside rounds, he flits from chair to chair, rather than manning a single station. Here awaits the actress/model Carey Lowell, a rangy, amiable woman with a damp shag in need of reshaping. Fekkai dismisses the idea that he is primarily a lover of layers. "No, it's not only layers and it's not only bobs. I'm attracted to the word 'horizon' – the idea of wide-open possibilities. I do all kinds of work for all kinds of people. I'm not into trends. You must always listen to and observe carefully the hair's texture, and never impose an idea on hair that it is incapable of receiving. Otherwise, you are giving a woman a style she cannot duplicate at home." In the split second before Fekkai initiates a cut, he sees in his mind's eye the "silhouette or outline" that he wishes to achieve, and from there he "plays with the hair" until the vision is realized. For Carey, a client of five years, he aims for something "very mobile, not too flat, very soft." A blur of motion, he rushes from side to side, inscribing a semicircle around her as he snips. He interrupts this dance of the scissors only to discuss whether the little tail of hair at the nape of her neck should stay or go. It comes off.

[5:00 PM] "After 11 years you're asking me what I want?" says Cynthia Nachmani, the Head of Education at the Museum of Modern Art, and the wife of psychoanalyst Dr. Gilead Nachmani. One of his earliest clients – "She got me just off the boat at the Bruno Dessange Salon," Fekkai says – Nachmani has made him the family hairdresser. "My husband comes here, and so does my 15-year-old son. He thinks Frederic is *the* man, and the salon is *the* coolest place to be. Everyone loves Frederic. He's very gentle." So what *does* Cynthia want? "Something easy to work with. It's important not to have to think about hair."

[5:15 PM] "I'm going to give you something very glamorous, with a swing. And a bit of an angle above the right eye." The lady whom Fekkai is addressing, "a dark-eyed, dark-haired, red-lipsticked woman," is, in his judgment, an ideal candidate for a blunt cut. "She needs definite structure and definite shape. But not severity. I don't do severe. It's not flattering. There's too much severity in

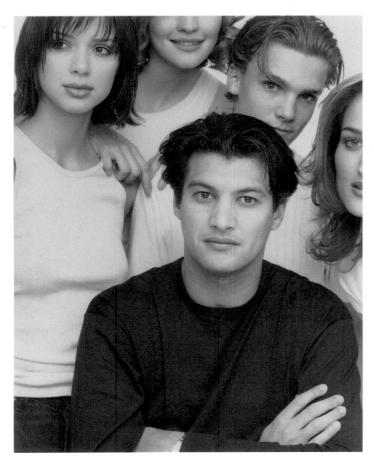

Frederic Fekkai and models, photographed by Didier Malige for Frederic Fekkai

Hairstory

STYLIST: *Frederic Fekkai*
SALON ADDRESS: *The Frederic Fekkai Beauty Center (for women),*
and L'Homme de Frederic Fekkai (for men), Bergdorf Goodman,
754 Fifth Avenue, New York City
PLACE OF BIRTH: *Aix-en-Provence, France*
FIRST JOB: *A stylist at The Bruno Dessange Salon, 1983*
TRADEMARKS: *Geometric cuts; His good looks; Flirting with clients*

Photograph by Didier Malige for Frederic Fekkai

"I set Katy's hair with big rollers, sprayed with volumizer then gently brushed out."

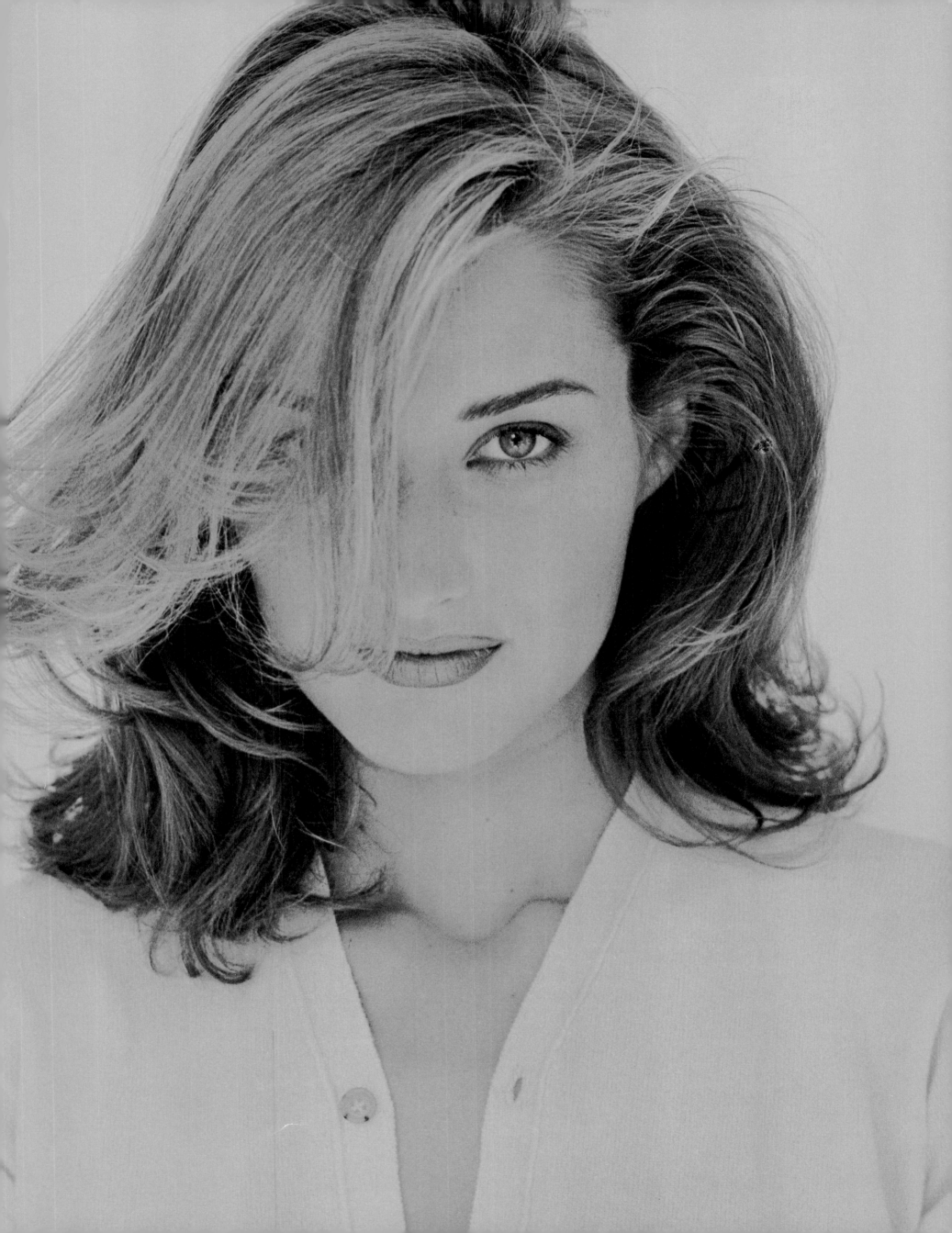

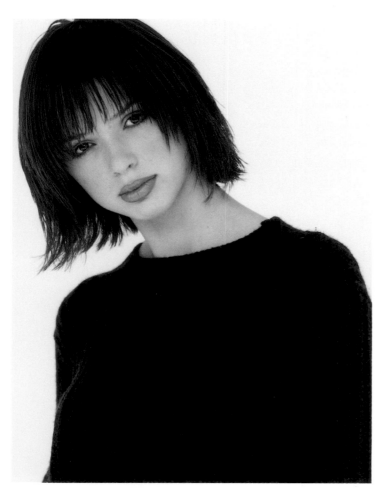

Photograph by Didier Malige for Frederic Fekkai

"This is a very basic look: It is a combination of a structured shape with lots of layers to keep the hair separated and wispy. I applied gel texturizer and finishing cream for shine."

our lives already. People need softness." The style agreed upon, the two of them break into familiar chatter about their respective Hamptons houses. (Nobody buries her nose in a magazine while Fekkai twiddles and clips.) The hairdresser, it emerges, has been so busy he hasn't visited his Long Island retreat for five months. Both vow to take full advantage of their second homes next summer. Fekkai, it is clear, lives a life similar to — and maybe sometimes better than — those of many of his clients. In fact, he socializes with them both in town and in the Hamptons. "How can you avoid it?" he asks rhetorically. When he's finished her trim, he asks the woman to shake her still-moist head. Disseminating a mist of droplets, her sleek, dark tresses languidly rearrange themselves. "I have to observe how the hair behaves," Fekkai notes. "Hair does what it wants." Pleased with her reflection in the mirror, the client adds, "No one can balance my hair the way Frederic does." Before proceeding to the next client, Fekkai states the obvious: "I really love this work. That's what keeps me going."

[5:30 PM] Fekkai assumes his position behind the chair of a stout, short-haired woman, a Midwestern heiress who commutes between Manhattan and her hometown. Inspired by a magazine story about Fekkai giving his son, Alexander, his first haircut, they exchange pleasantries about their children. Fekkai apparently has indelibly engraved in his memory the details of each customer's personal and professional lives — a task made easier by the fact that 80% of his clients are regulars. "I'm changing everything slightly to make the hair fuller around the face," Fekkai

announces, pulling up sections of hair to meet his scissors. "I'm following the shape of the head. With the haircut, it's always an evolution. Otherwise I get bored." The woman, a Fekkai follower for six years, smiles in assent. "We'd both get bored," she says.

[5:45 PM] Now it's time for Marla Maples Trump, who has been attracting glances with her gracious, expectant show-biz smile. Fekkai has not altered his schedule to accommodate her, however; he is the one star of this show. Marla drawls sweetly, "After five years Frederic and I finally got up the nerve to shorten my hair by five inches. I called all my friends, and discussed it with my husband, and they all told me 'no, don't do it.' But I listened to Frederic. I felt so happy, and so liberated. When I came home, Donald changed his mind. He loved my attitude — I felt so young and sexy! My new haircut is much better with the baby, and much better for my career. Frederic has gotten very creative with me." Fekkai explains his motivation for the change: "When her hair was longer, Marla looked too much like a Barbie doll. I've given her a modern twist — she's no longer a cliché." With only an anonymous smock and wet fringes of blonde hair to set off her valentine-heart face, Marla looks arrestingly beautiful. It's easy to see why Fekkai is loathe to overwhelm her pert, delicate features with heavy cascades of hair. Like an abstract artist analyzing a painting's composition, Fekkai demonstrates how every angle, line, and curve of his haircut is calculated to echo, reinforce, and draw out the arcs and planes of Marla's graceful face. The layers swoop along an eyebrow, tilt to meet the jawbone, dive into a

Kelly Killeron, photographed by Didier Malige for Frederic Fekkai

"I've always loved hair that is primarily one length, but with layers and a faux fringe. It's a simple, wash-and-wear kind of style, yet there is tremendous movement in the hair. I applied some texturizing balm to prevent it looking 'fly-away' and to maintain body."

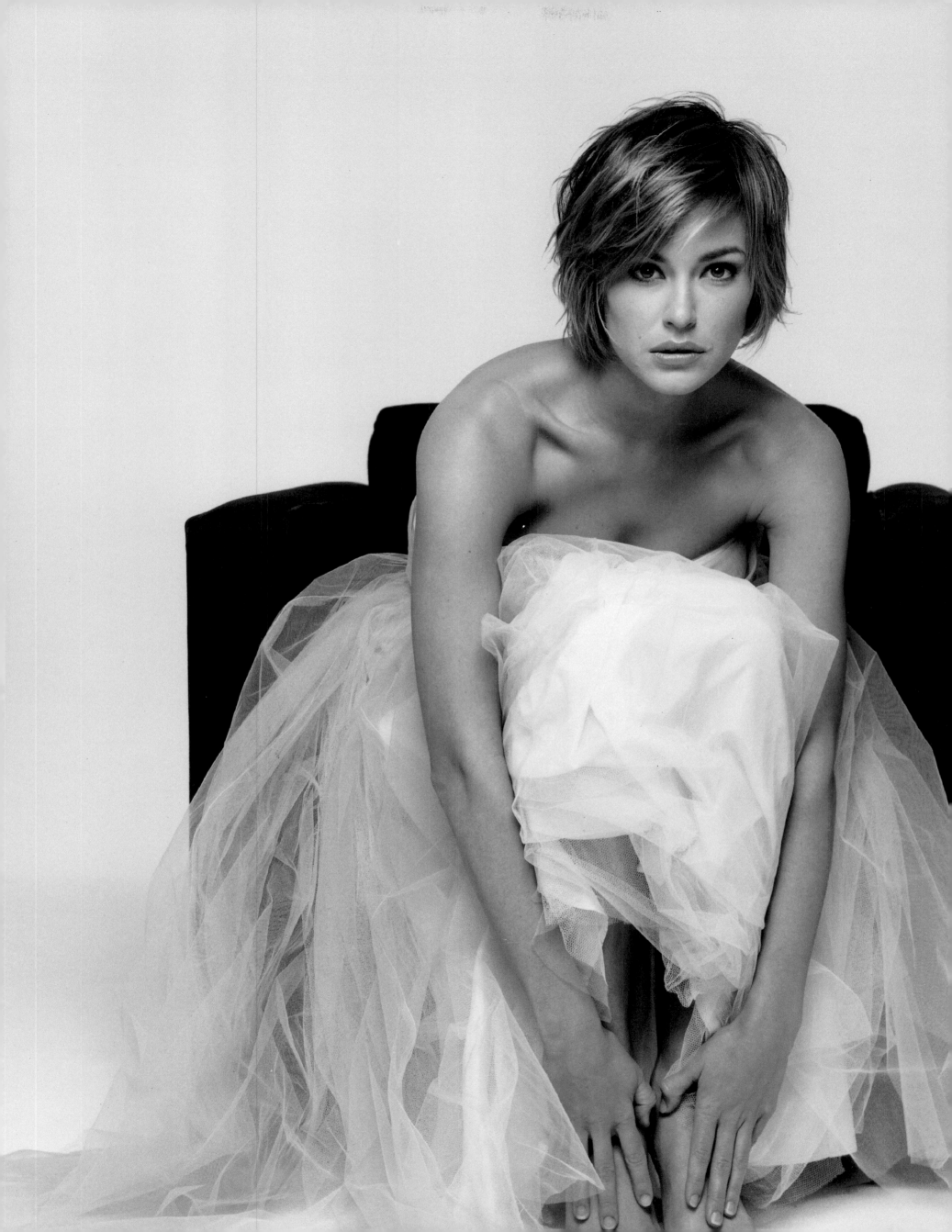

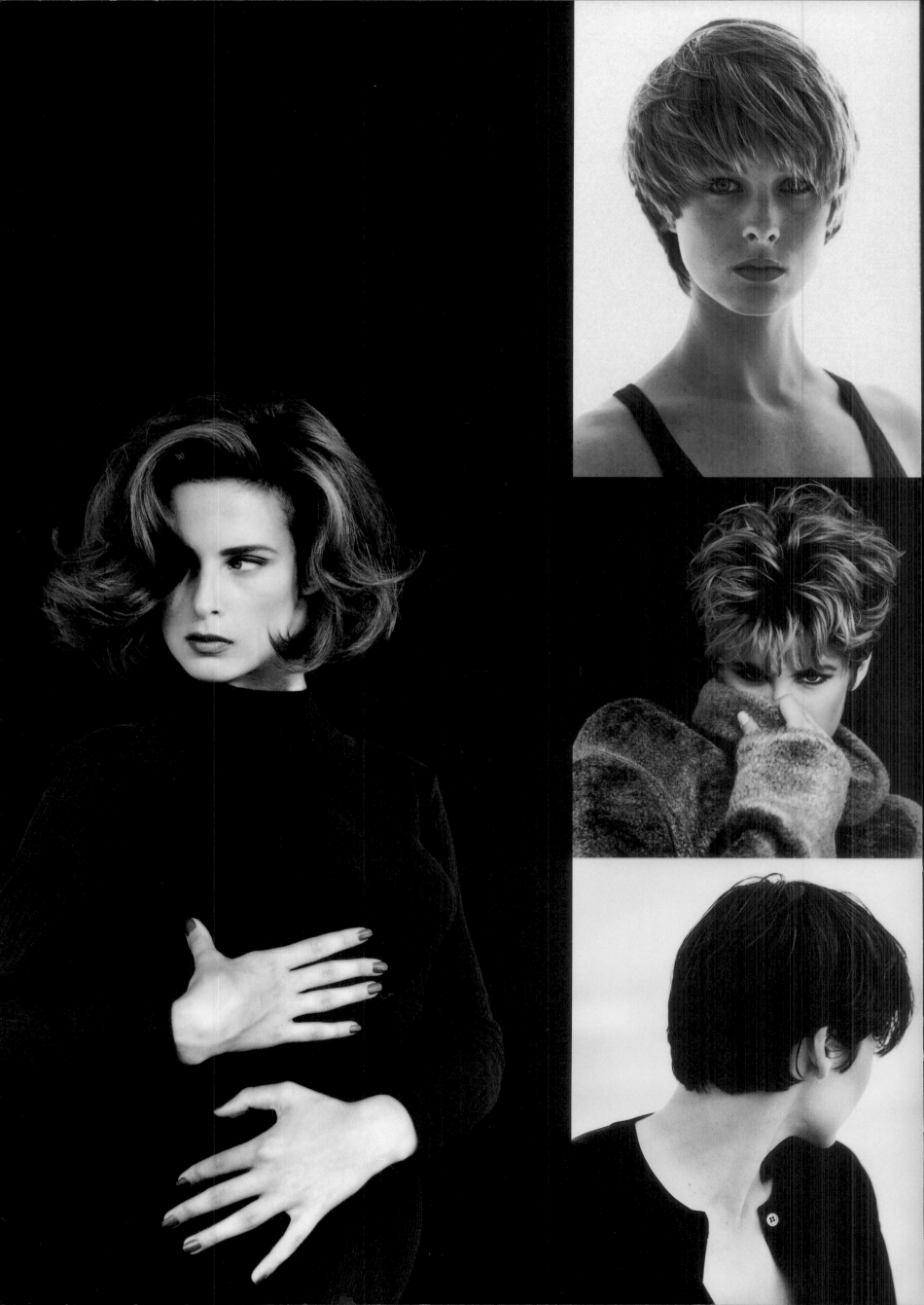

cheekbone, trail along a collarbone – a Kandinsky rendered in hair. The studied resonances between facial traits and strands, however, are much less evident once her locks are dried and puffed up by a blower. It's not surprising that Trump himself forgoes the artistic Fekkai treatment, preferring instead to be shorn by the family barber. "But Donald and Frederic have a project that they're working on together. May I say what it is?" Marla asks. Fekkai's only retort is to elongate his fleshy lips into a silent, sphinx-like grin.

[6:00 PM] A slightly agitated, snub-nosed woman is lifting her long, sandy tresses to expose a small bald patch just above her left ear. Fekkai peers and pokes, while the two murmur discreetly about hair loss, shaving, and dermatology. "I think we need privacy for this," Fekkai says deferentially.

[6:15 PM] When Susan Feigenson, Vice President of Merchandising for a men's sportswear company, first surrendered her head to Frederic Fekkai, she overcame the greatest phobia of her life. "I was completely, utterly paranoid about getting my hair cut. Then someone I knew who had the same fear went to Frederic, and I knew I could do it too. I was gripping the table in front of me for dear life. But I got over it and now I will never go to anyone else." Needless to say, Fekkai has no wild designs upon Susan's hair, today or ever. What he gives her, he says, is "a classic, nice bob. If

you layered Susan's full, curly hair, it would get frizzy, difficult to control. It is important always to have the upper hand with hair." With a blunt cut, he says, the general shape of the head, rather than individual features, is taken into account. But simplicity does not come easily. "The blunt cut is one of the most difficult to achieve," Fekkai says. "You have to study the technical aspects of the hair. How is it going to react when it passes over the shoulders? How will it respond at the back of the neck? The beauty of a bob comes from shape, balance, and proportion." Susan, meanwhile, has transferred some of her anxieties onto another hair-related subject. "Frederic, is it a bad idea to come here at the end of the day like I always do? Aren't you bored already by this hour?" No, no, insists Fekkai, *au contraire*. In fact, because he has such passion for his work, his enthusiasm actually increases throughout the day. "A neurosurgeon friend of mine told me the same thing about his work," says the hairstylist.

[6:30 – 8:30 PM] The clients who fill the last slots in his appointment book (among them Dominique Browning, the new Editor-in-Chief of *House & Garden* magazine) should be grateful to learn they will be getting Fekkai at peak form. For when Fekkai cuts, he penetrates – if not exactly into the brain, then deep into the psyche.

Facing page, left: *"High Glamour. This is a set done with big Velcro rollers, after applying volumizer spray to the roots. Once the hair was dry, I relaxed it a little with a hairbrush and hairdryer, so it would look bouncy and not too rigid."*

Right top: *"A Beatles-inspired cut, but modernized. Androgynous and sexy."* **Model: Julia Hine**

Right middle: *"This style is achieved by applying gel to wet hair, then finger waving and pinning the hair. Once the hair was dry, I loosened the curls with my fingers and cold air from a hairdryer."*

Right bottom: *"Carey has beautiful bone structure and magnificent eyes. I cut her hair short with a lot of layers and no part for this very sexy wash-and-go style."* **Model: Carey Lowell**

Below left: *"This is a 'Gavroche' kind of look, achieved by spraying the roots with volumizer, blow-drying straight and smooth with a definite part to accentuate the asymmetric feel."*

Below middle: *"What you see here is the cut only. I towel-dried the hair, combed through a very light conditioner and asked Carey to simply shake her head."* **Model: Carey Lowell**

Right: *"I gave Farrah a great, young look – it requires no maintenance. In fact, it looks better unkempt."* **Model: Farrah Summerford**

All photographs on this page were photographed by Didier Malige for Frederic Fekkai.

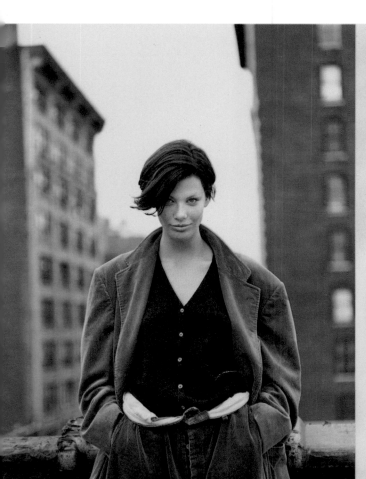
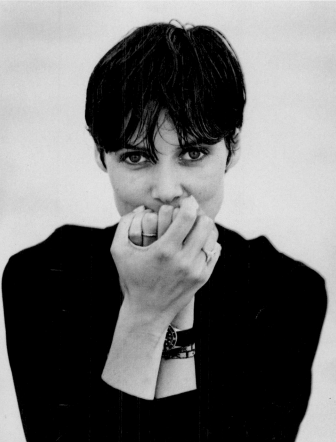
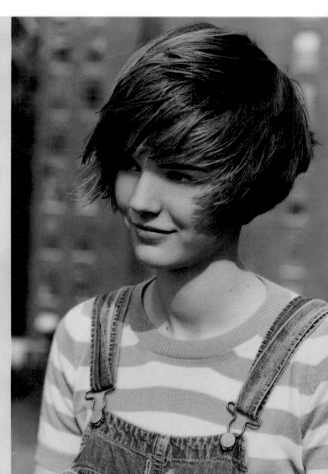

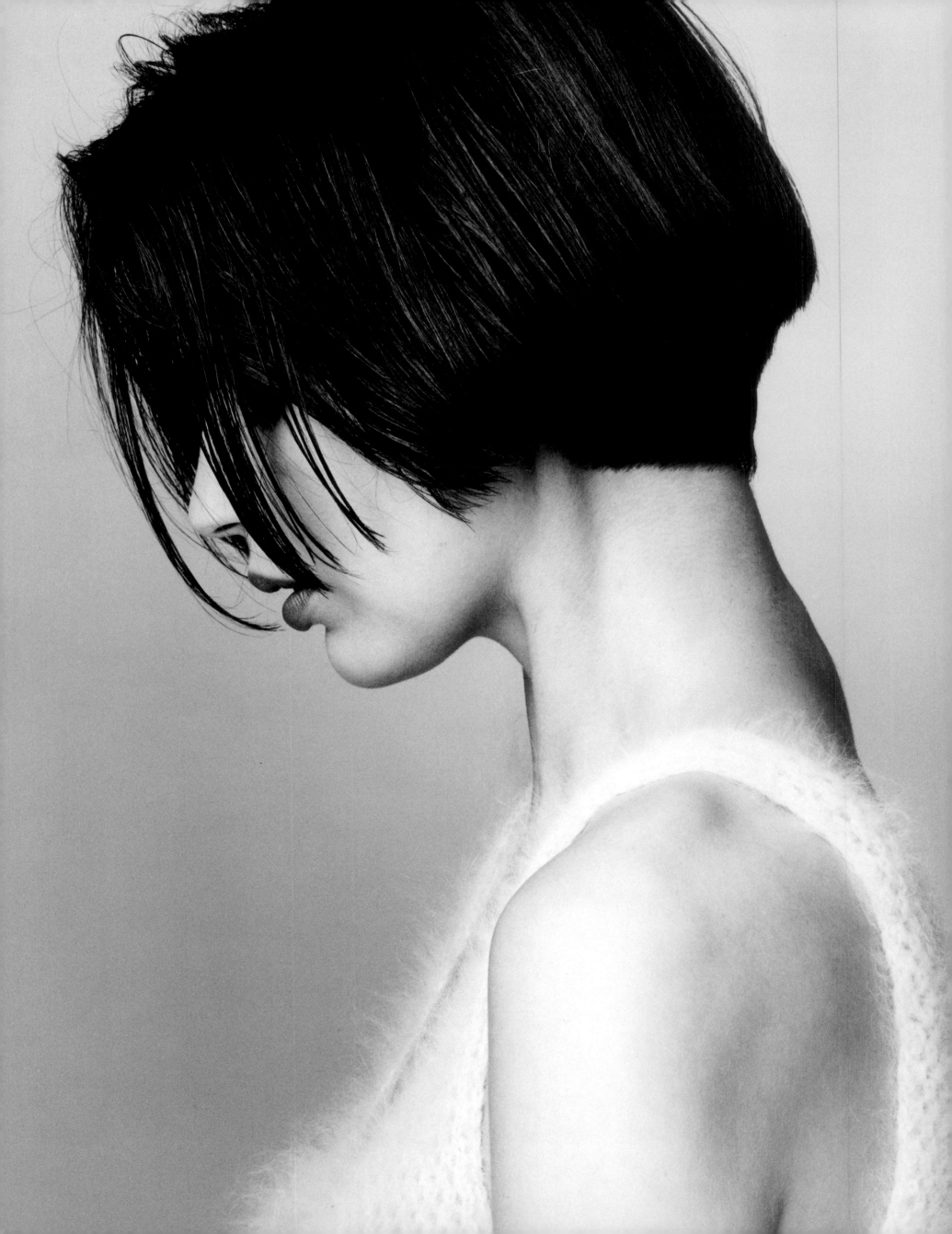

Likes

CUT:
working *with* the natural texture of the hair – not against it
choosing a cut that fits the client's personality and profession
clients who stand up during the cut

COLOR:
natural-looking color

STYLE:
understated chic

TREATMENT:
using his ten-product line

Dislikes

CUT:
cuts that are too short on top and too long in back
spiked hair
wedge cuts
cuts that are too trendy

COLOR:
ash blonde that looks green
covering up gray

STYLE:
unnecessary perms
the wet-gel look
high hair on an oval face
large hair ornaments like bows and ribbons
hair fragrance

TREATMENT:
products that are tested on animals

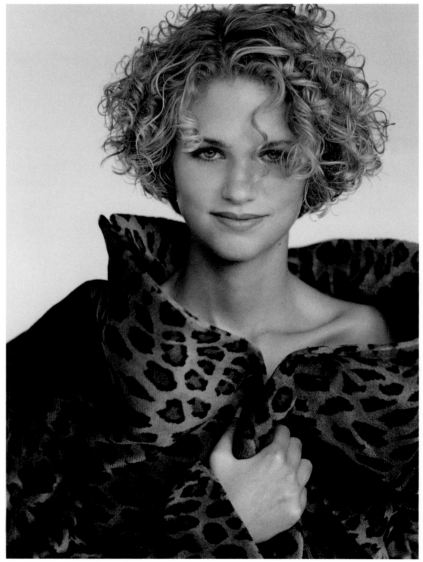

Sullivan, photographed by Didier Malige for Frederic Fekkai

"Here I applied a cream/texturizer/gel throughout the hair and scrunched it up with a diffuser/dryer."

Louisa, photographed by Didier Malige for Frederic Fekkai

"With a cut like this, it is important to keep the hair in sharp style using gel at the roots and a finishing cream to make it stringy and shiny."

Photograph by Mark Babushkin. Courtesy of L'Oréal Technique Professionelle
©L'Oréal Technique Professionelle

"I wanted a glamorous look, so I first applied gel mixed with sculpting lotion to the roots to get body, then blew the hair dry. I supported sections of the hair with clips to achieve smoother waves and the flip."

Do's & Don'ts

Get a hairstyle that represents you.

Let your look/hairstyle be distinctive.

Don't overstyle. Avoid too much teasing, hairspray.

Work *with* your hair, not against it.

Fashion trends should influence your style, not dictate it.

Your hairstyle should be realistic, interesting.

Don't let your hair get damaged or overprocessed.

Avoid stereotypical looks.

Have a definite style, but not necessarily all the time. Vary it.

Challenge your stylist with ideas.

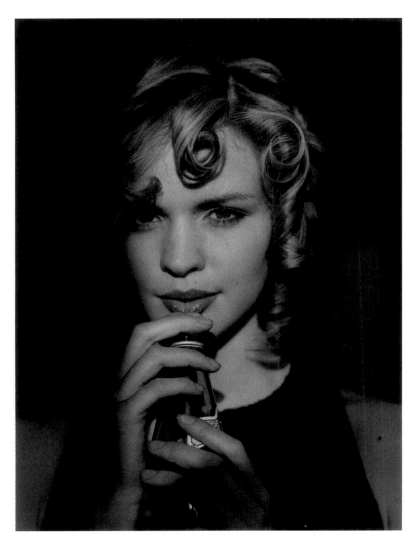

Photograph by Didier Malige for Frederic Fekkai

"Having applied gel to wet hair, I pin-curled it, let it dry, and left it."

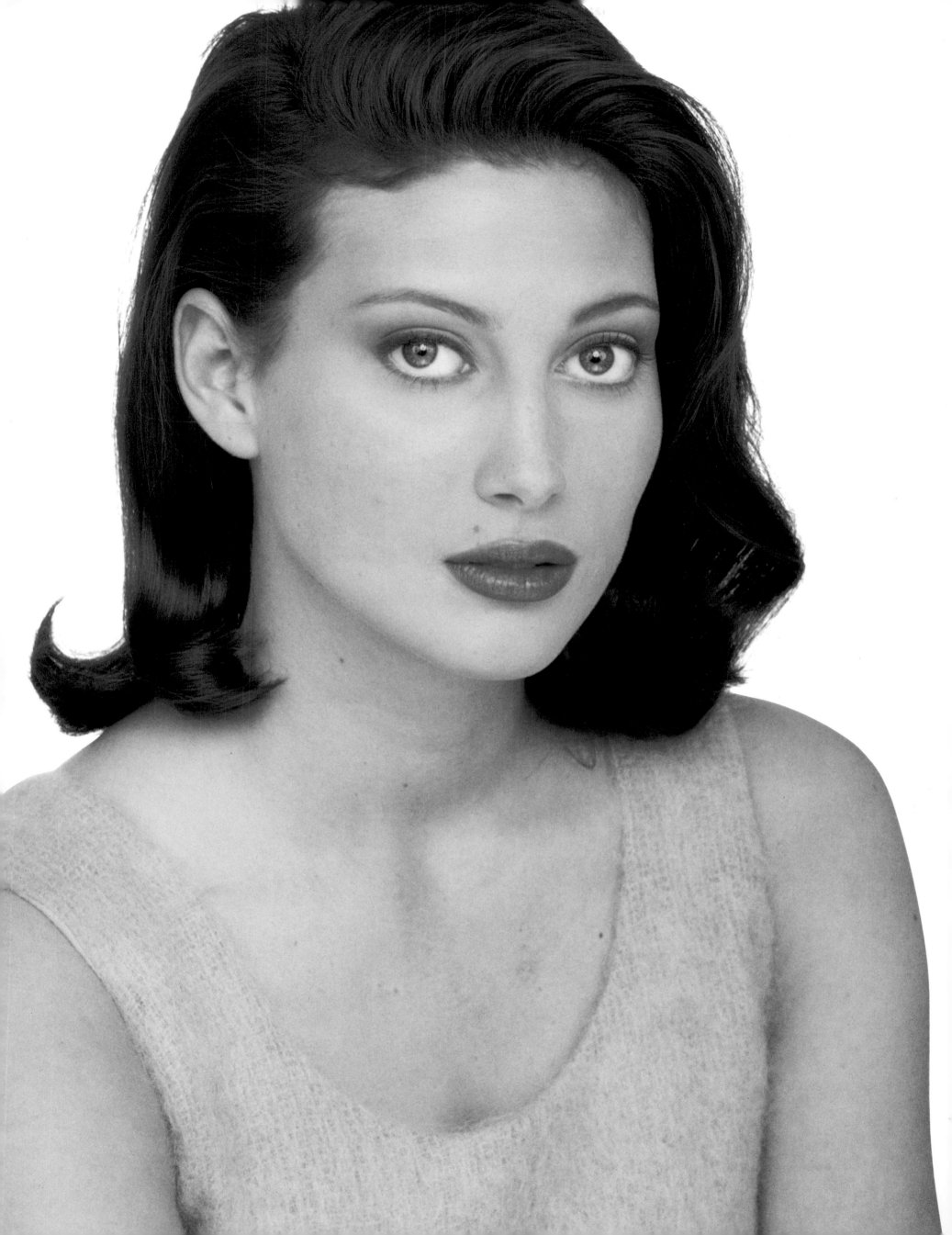

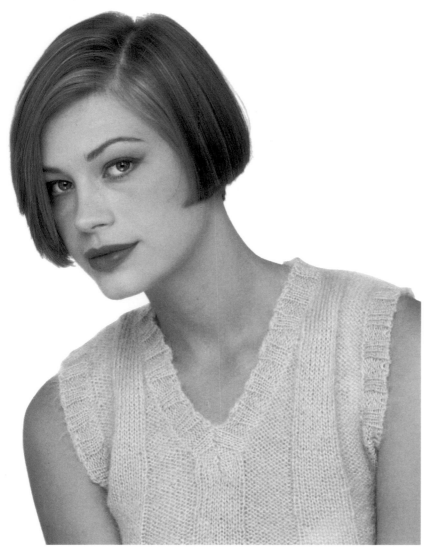

Clients

Jodie Foster

Peter Gabriel

Steffi Graf

Twyla Tharp

Mariah Carey

John F. Kennedy, Jr.

Barbra Streisand

Marla Maples Trump

Kelly Klein

Jessica Lange

Photograph by Mark Babushkin. Courtesy of L'Oréal Technique Professionelle.
©L'Oréal Technique Professionelle

"This graphic, smooth look can be achieved by blow-drying straight and flat, and then applying silicone for shine."

Photograph by Didier Malige for Frederic Fekkai

"Very messy, very chic, very feminine."

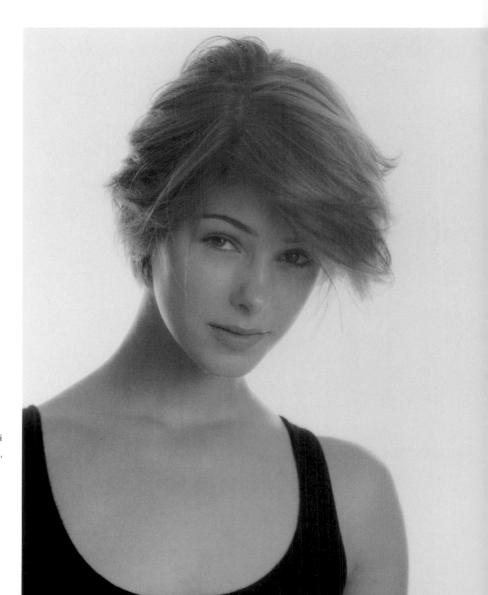

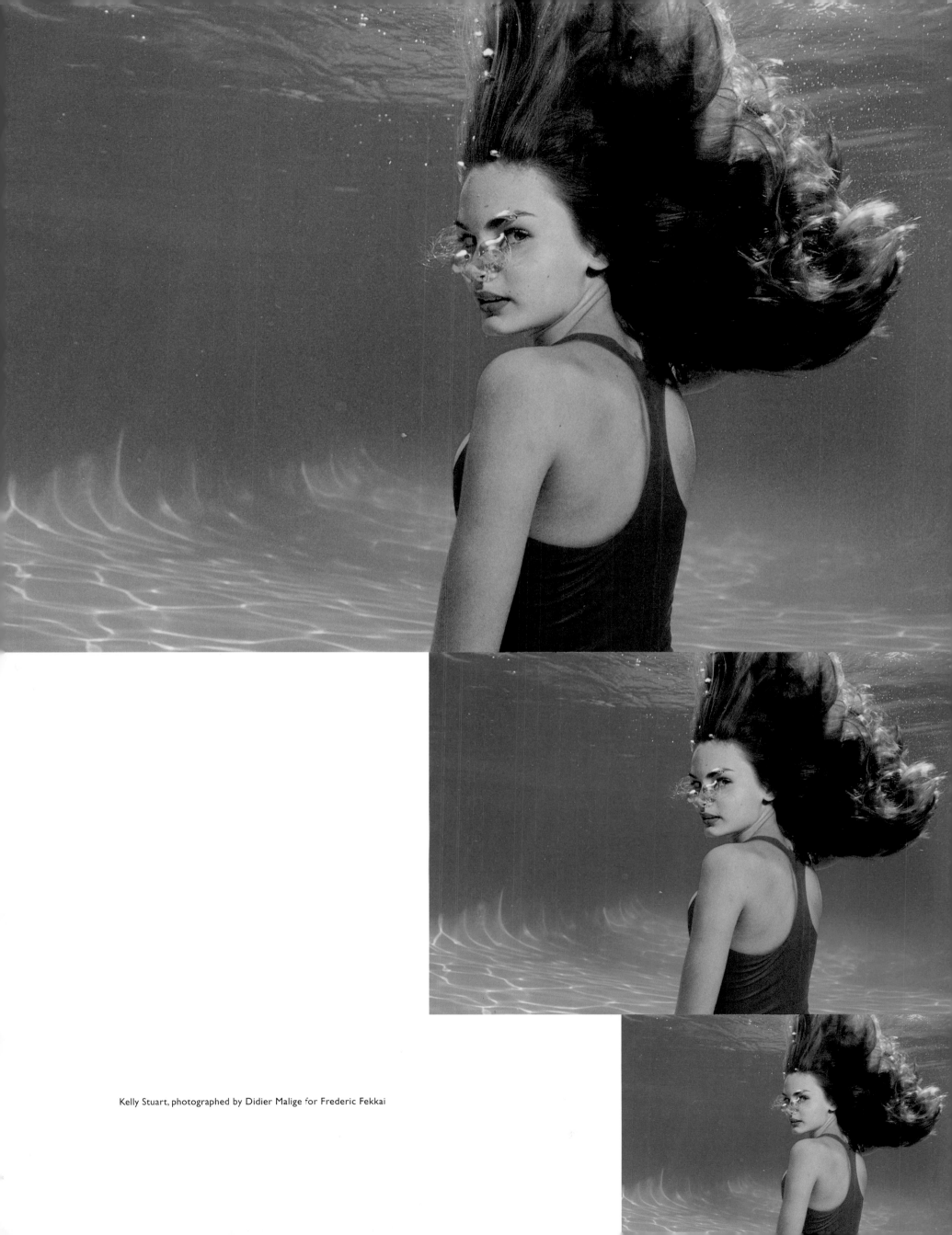

Kelly Stuart, photographed by Didier Malige for Frederic Fekkai

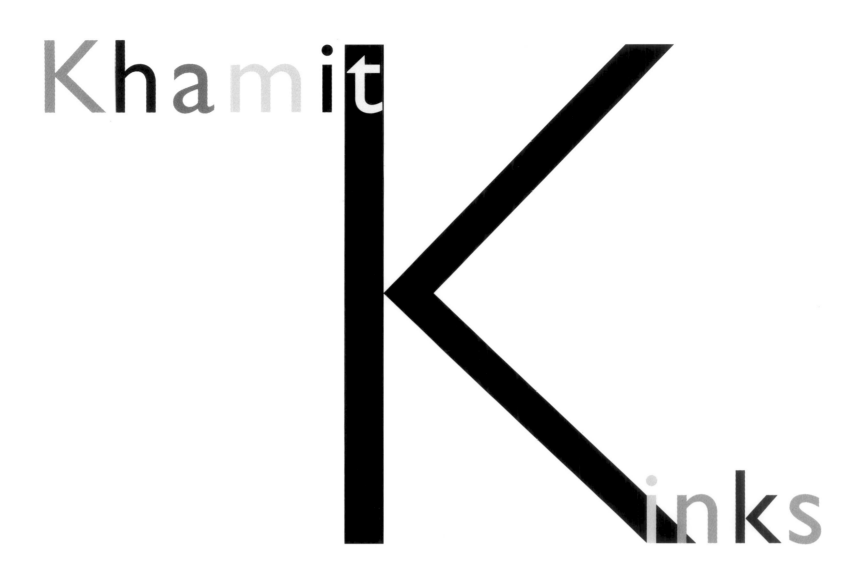

Khamit Kinks

Braids and Bravado

On Halsey Street in Bedford-Stuyvesant, Brooklyn, a neighborhood better known for hard knocks than for aesthetic refinements, stands a temple known as Khamit Kinks, consecrated to the arcane art of African braiding. Tucked away on the basement level of an 1880s brownstone, the salon has an atmosphere both extemporaneous and timeless. The walls are painted sugary purple – the color of candied violets – and the antique wooden vanities, acquired from a local dealer, don't match. Gliding regally through these cloistered premises are the exotically named priestesses of Khamit Kinks, their hair magnificently arranged into headdress-like coifs, their bodies robed in stately African gowns. The proprietress comes forward to introduce herself as "Annu Prestonia. Annu is a name from ancient Khamit," she explains. "Khamit is what Egypt was originally called before the Greeks. Khamit, by the way, is pronounced 'cammit,' dammit! 'Kinks' refers to the texture of our hair. The salon's name came to me in a dream." Annu's more conventionally named partner, Ruth Sinclair – "she's the creative director of the company and I'm the technical director" – tends the second Khamit Kinks salon, established four years ago in Atlanta. The two women, whose work is regularly featured in *Essence* and other magazines, have also launched a line of emulsifying oils to nourish and cleanse black hair. "It tends to be very dry, the opposite of Caucasian hair, which is usually oily," Annu says. Khamit Kinks is so preeminent on the black hair circuit that for the past six years it has garnered most of the major awards at annual braiders' competitions in Washington, Atlanta, and New York. At her salon and in photographers' studios, Annu has worked on the heads of Angela Bassett, Angela Davis, Iman, Queen Latifah, Joie and Spike Lee (for his movie *Crooklyn*), Beverly Peele, Stevie Wonder, and Oprah Winfrey (who will not release any pictures of herself in Khamit Kinks braids). "She asked for a style that she could wear while swimming," Annu says.

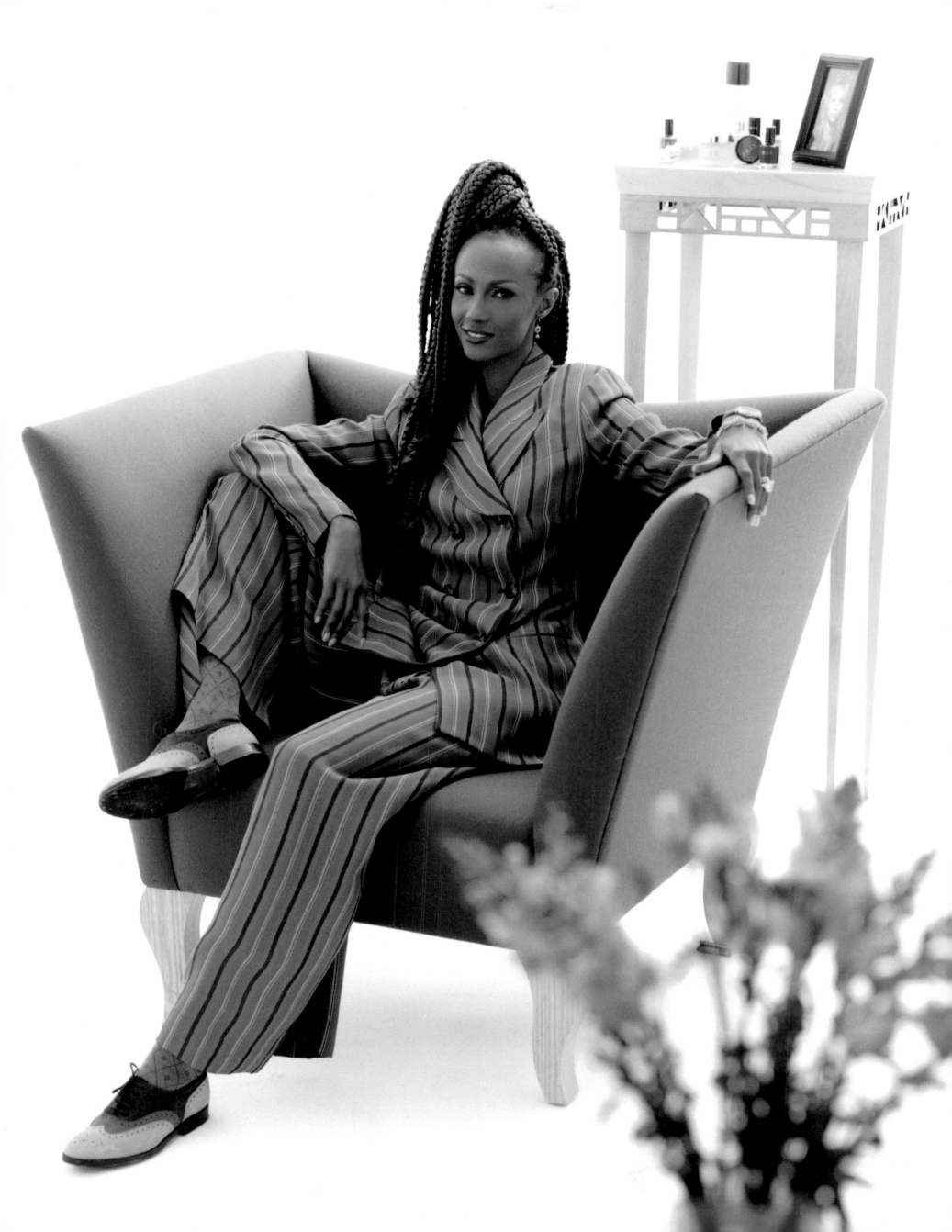

One of Annu's initiates is Amma, Khamit's specialist in thread wraps — a labor-intensive process that involves coiling thread tightly around numerous long sections of hair, then piling the sections up into a sculptural, serpentine nexus that rests on the head like a free-form crown. Amma — whose own splendid helmet of meticulously groomed dreadlocks gives her the mysterious dignity of a sphinx — is thread wrapping just the front portion of the hair of a woman named Merisa. Simultaneously, Annu is braiding the back into attenuated, tentacle-like plaits. The resulting hairdo, Annu explains, is called the "High-Low." Every Khamit Kinks creation comes with a name (Georgia Peach and Nefertiti are two more examples), as well it should — each is a fantastical work of art deserving of a title. "No style ever turns out the same way twice," Annu states proudly. "Everybody's hair is different, and so is every head shape." Adds Amma, a self-taught braider with 20 years of experience, "Most clients let me do what I want."

Merisa, whose tribal-print dress is protected by an iridescent purple smock, will have to sit for two to three hours while Annu's and Amma's fingers fly. Khamit's most elaborate braiding procedures can take more than eight hours. In addition to warning clients that profanities, intoxicants, and smoking are against house rules, the salon's brochure advises customers to pack books, paperwork, and lunch because of the protracted length of the braiding sessions. ("Order lunch in?" Annu crows. "You're in the wrong 'hood!") Khamit's prolonged, concentrated, and skillful attentions do not come cheap. The average Khamit do — Merisa's High-Low or a headful of short Senegalese Twists (supple two-strand plaits similar in appearance to licorice sticks) — hovers around $200. A nonrefundable cash, money-order, or credit card deposit must be paid in advance of all appointments.

The salon's "most expensive creation," Annu says, "is below-the-shoulder fake locks. Many people are too impatient to grow long locks. They want them immediately. It takes six to eight hours, with two, three, even four stylists working at once" — at a cost of around $600. Taking into account labor and time, this is not a bad deal. Amma says she typically works on only two to four clients a day, and a coiffure such as Merisa's High-Low will hold up for about two months.

Most of the styles, Merisa's included, are executed with artificial hair extensions imported from Asia. Synthetic hair is "more uniform, more tameable, and doesn't change with the weather," Annu says. Currently, Khamit Kinks' most popular style is Silky Dreads, a luxurious lock variant made from shiny hair extensions. Both Annu's and Amma's locks, however, are entirely their own. Annu's, unlike her colleague's, are short, bleached ("with Clairol") to a rusty gold, and pin-curled. (The salon will color, but not relax, hair; cutting is "minimal," and weaves — which result in the straight, false hair often seen on Naomi Campbell — are antithetical, of course, to a salon named Kinks.) "This is my second set of locks," Annu reports. "My first ones grew so long and heavy they gave me a headache."

Braiding (a general term used to cover all Khamit's methods), Annu recalls, is "something I learned from my mother" during her Norfolk, Virginia, upbringing. "Children always wore their hair braided as a way of helping their hair grow. Braiding was definitely always in the culture, but as an African tradition it had been looked on as something negative, not suitable for adults." With the Black Power movement of the 60s, braids began to resurface on adults — at first as a way to set Afros. "I remember we used to braid guys' hair after basketball games, because their Afros would

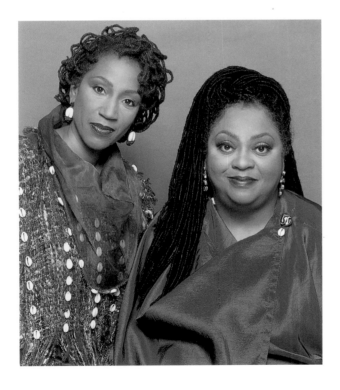

Hairstory

STYLISTS: *Annu Prestonia and Ruth Sinclair*

SALON ADDRESS: *107a Halsey Street, Brooklyn, New York*

PLACE OF BIRTH: *Portsmouth, Virginia; Raleigh, North Carolina*

FIRST JOB: *In a record store; The Automat*

TRADEMARKS: *Outstanding quality; Definition and execution of braids*

Annu Prestonia and Ruth Sinclair, photographed by Wayne Summerlin for Khamit Kinks

Queen Latifah, photographed by Timothy White for *Essence*. Courtesy *Essence*

"Two months before it appeared on the cover of Essence, *Ruth Sinclair of the Atlanta Khamit Kinks designed this style, which she named the Queen Latifah, with the performer in mind."*

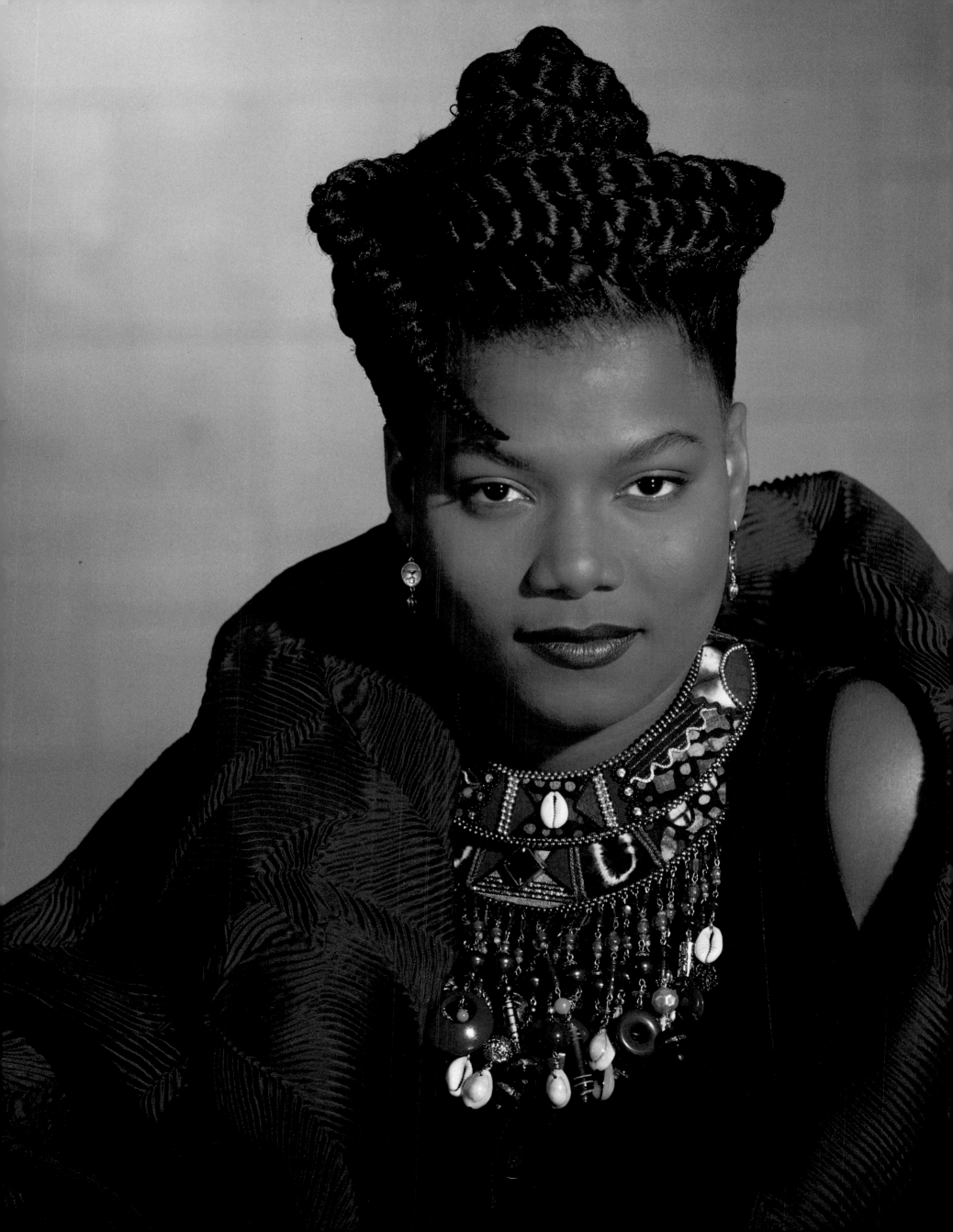

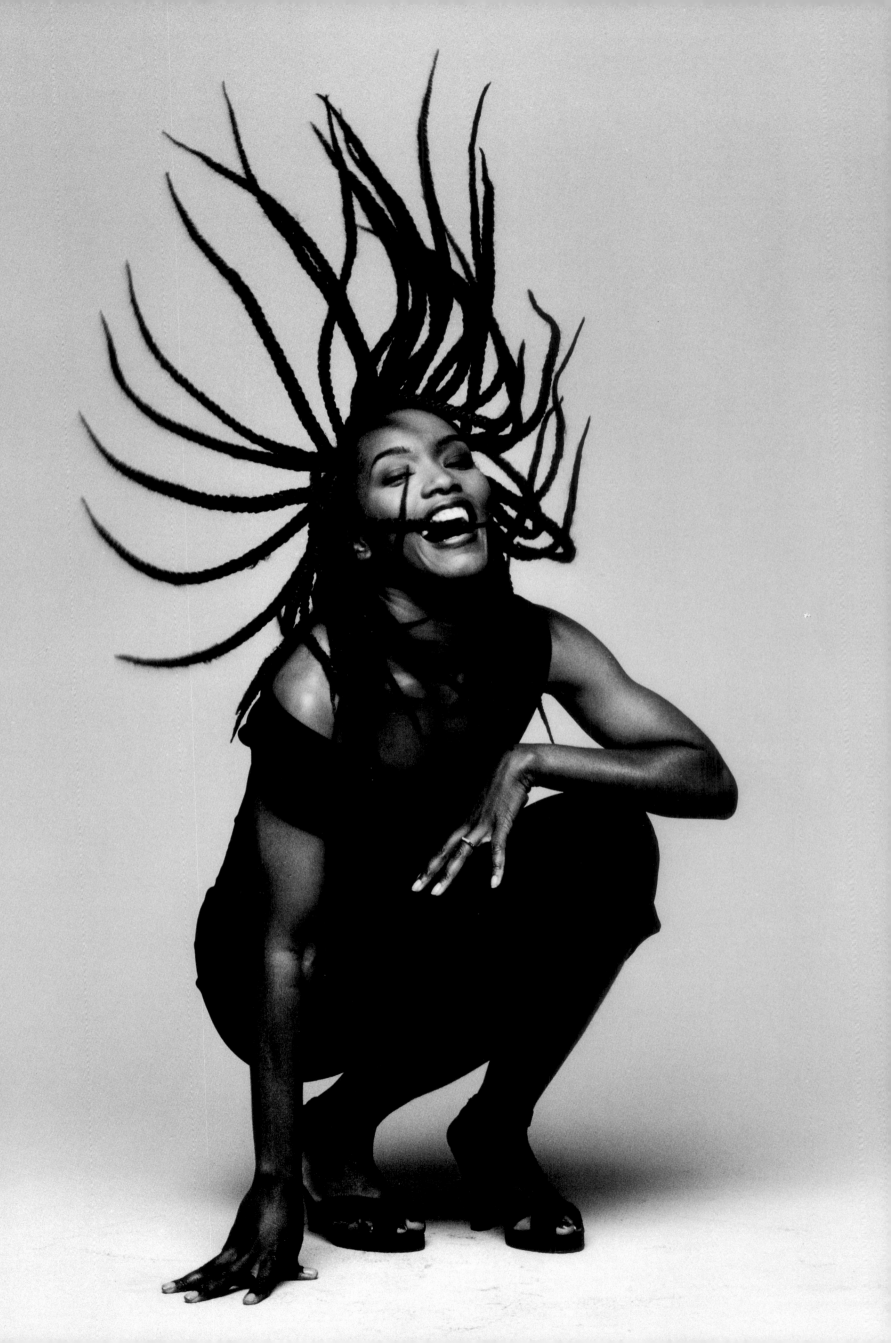

"Here, Angela Bassett's extra-long Casamas braids create movement and sensuality. Though a stylist was present, it's clear that Angela makes this style work through the sheer force of her personality. When Annu first saw the Casamas braid in Senegal, West Africa, she was mesmerized by its beauty. In the States, small, tiny braids were all the rage; Annu had never seen such a finely crafted large braid: tightly woven, tapered to a tee, with a weave representing the perfection of a craft. The Casamas had uniformity, flow, and energy. It stood out like no other braid."

shrink from sweating," Annu says. "And women used to incorporate braiding with their Afros, to make patterns." As Afros waned in popularity, braiding and locks supplanted them as symbols of black pride. Interestingly, what Americans call French braids are in France referred to as *tresses africaines*.

In a chair at the far end of the Khamit salon, a stylist named Marva has begun giving a client a combination of thread wraps and Goddess braids, extravagant cornrows as fat as soft pretzels. Annu, meanwhile, is finishing off Merisa's braids with the aid of a burning white candle, held securely in a glass dish. By singeing their tips, Annu seals the braids so they will not unravel — one advantage of the extension's man-made fiber. Then she deftly runs the flame along the length of each braid, a ritual that allows each long twist to curve seductively toward the face.

The candlestick ceremony completed, Annu, a woman with entrepreneurial vision, pauses to contemplate the future. "My dream is to open a full-service salon — a kind of Red Door for black women. We can get facials, manicures, and massages done at any spa, but not our hair. I also want to make and sell more products. I'd especially like to produce educational materials — a coffee-table book and how-to videos. People already call me from Idaho and Alaska asking for video instructions on braiding. In Africa, the most time-consuming hairstyles were reserved only for royalty. But we're all queens now!"

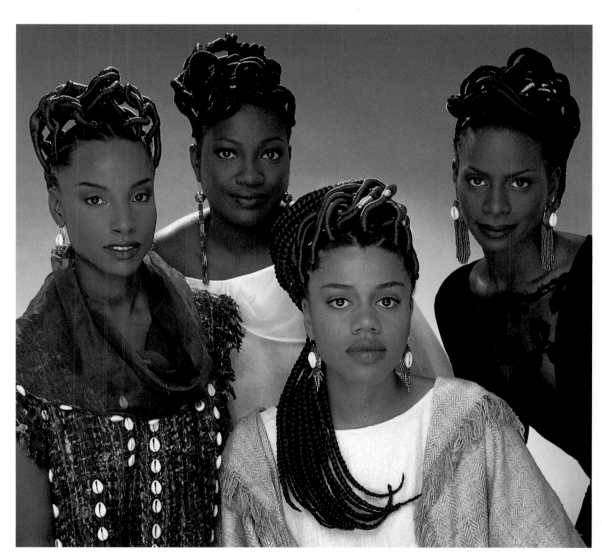

Chanette Peoples, Marva White-Walters, Leslie Cognalatti, and Roxanna Floyd, photographed by Preston Phillips for Khamit Kinks

"The scalp patterns are part of the geometry of the hairstyle. The model in front is wearing a combination of thread wraps and Casamas. The braids curl under because of the closeness of the weave, which is a necessity for Casamas braids. The model at the right rear has chosen thread wraps to go over her natural locks for a change of pace. Thread wraps are styled to resemble crowns, thus emulating the look of royalty."

Likes

CUT:
Afrocentric geometric cuts from the late 80s

COLOR:
shades of red
off-black to amber

STYLE:
locks
hair worn with attitude and assurance
hair styled in accordance with the lifestyle of the client
hairstyles that demonstrate creativity
hairstyles that bring out the subtle dimensions
of the client's personality

TREATMENT:
henna
herbal rinses
hot oil treatments
cholesterol treatments
Khamit Kinks oils
natural shampoos that contain very few chemicals

Dislikes

CUT:
those given in the army
page boy

COLOR:
blue rinses on gray hair
stripped brass blonde with no color redeposited
bleaching
bright green and pink

STYLE:
"tried, dyed, laid to the side"
elaborate evening styles worn on ordinary days
short styles on round faces
long hair on long faces

TREATMENT:
any treatment that alters the natural structure of kinky
hair, e.g., chemical relaxers

Do's & Don'ts

Always be self-assured in your braid style; go to a professional who will consult with you on appropriate braid styles and will execute your style with skill, craftsmanship, and perfection. Don't settle for mediocrity. Natural and braided styles often cause discomfort in employment environments. An employer who forbids you to wear your hair in these styles is usually responding to one of two things: a tacky braid job, or the fact that you are not carrying off the hairstyle with class.

Don't pay for disappointment; if possible, go to the source. A braid salon whose portfolios are made up of clippings of other salons' work seldom executes a professional job.

Wear a braid style that fits the situation. There are hundreds of Afrocentric styles that are suitable for all occasions. With the help of a professional stylist, you can achieve daily, social, festive, and casual styles.

Refresh your braid style and reinforce the support needed at the hair line to keep the braids from breaking off. These styles have longevity, but that doesn't mean that daily grooming isn't required. Grooming and conditioning regimens should be scheduled regularly and should include moisture maintenance with natural oils, tying with a scarf, stationary styles for sleeping, wearing a shower cap for bathing, and shampooing and conditioning your braids. For long-term styles, a touch-up by the sixth week is important. This is achieved by removing the braids around the hair line and replacing them with freshly done braids.

No matter how good your braids look at the three-month period, regardless of how many compliments you're receiving, all braids should be removed by the fourth month unless you are planning to dreadlock your hair from that style. By the fourth month, braids are locked and removal can cause major hair breakage.

Photograph by John Peden for *Essence*. Courtesy *Essence*

"The Crawl — try this on your man for a hair-raising experience. Big Girl plaits, large slanted squares with braids extending below the waist, create animal magnetism. The secret to this hairstyle is not to weigh the scalp down with too many braids. Balance and distribution are important."

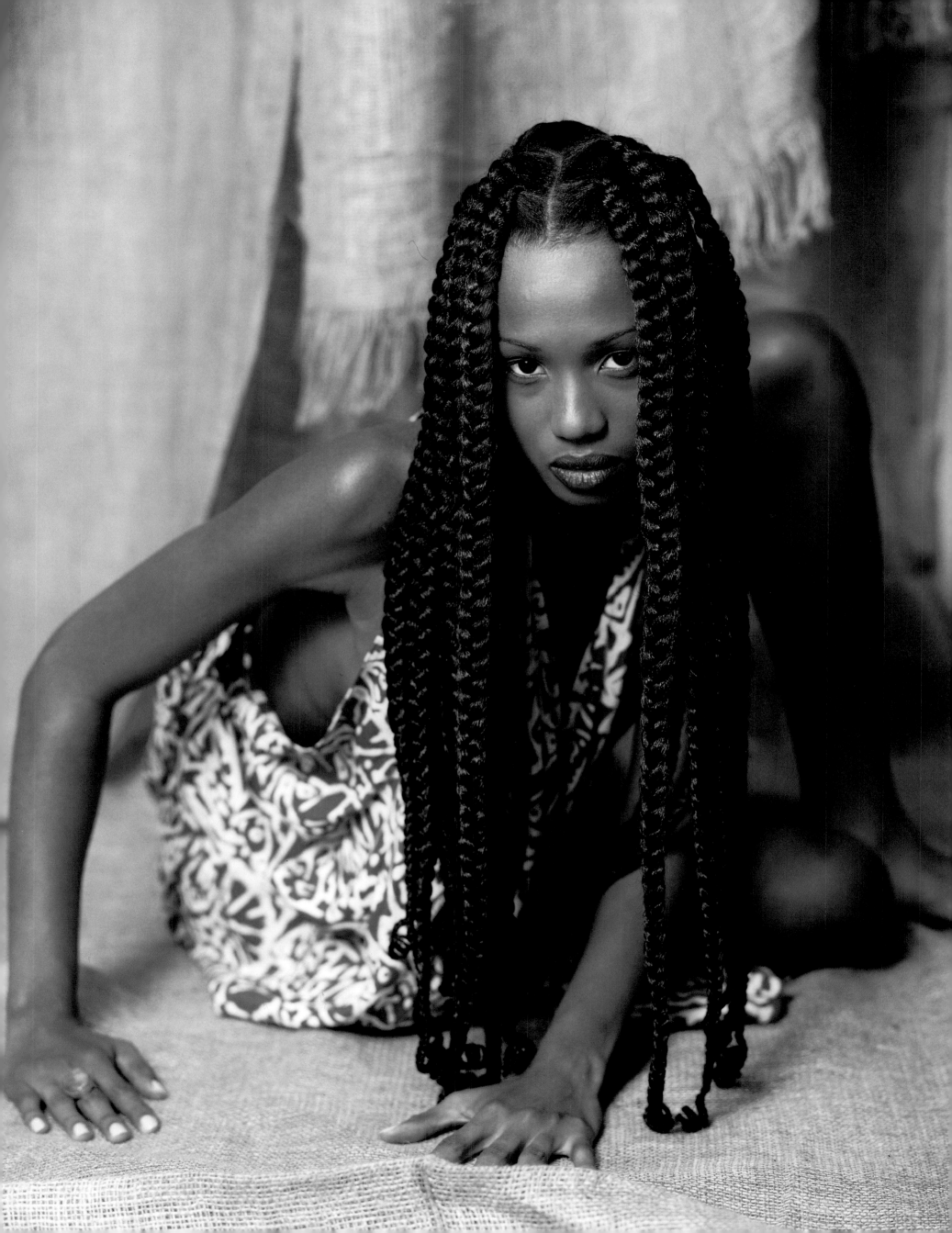

Misconceptions About Braids:

BRAIDING BREAKS THE HAIR. Braiding does not break the hair. However, improper application and/or removal of braids may cause breakage.

HUMAN HAIR IS BETTER THAN SYNTHETIC HAIR. They are both fine for braided styles. The difference is that human hair is more appropriate for looser styles, e.g., weaves. Synthetic hair is more appropriate for a more braided look. Synthetic hair holds the weave of the braid firmly and permanently. Human hair creeps, so the weave of the braid becomes lax as time goes by and the braid looks more like loose hair.

SYNTHETIC HAIR DAMAGES YOUR OWN HAIR. This is the biggest fallacy. Synthetic fiber does not damage your hair. If it did, the Kane-kelon Company, which makes the fiber, would not be a multi-million dollar industry. We're in the business of encouraging hair growth, so we would not use a fiber that harms the hair.

LOCKS ARE NOT GROOMED AND ARE UNCLEAN. Locked hair is groomed on a regular and continuous basis.

EXTENSIONS ARE WORN BY PEOPLE WHO ARE BALD OR HAVE LITTLE HAIR. Extensions create uniformity, fullness, longevity, and versatility. Most clients choose extensions for these reasons. Only 3% of our clients use extensions from lack of hair.

YOU CAN CREATE SHORT BRAIDS WHEN BRAIDING LONG HAIR. The long hair has to be cut first. . . . No miracles here!

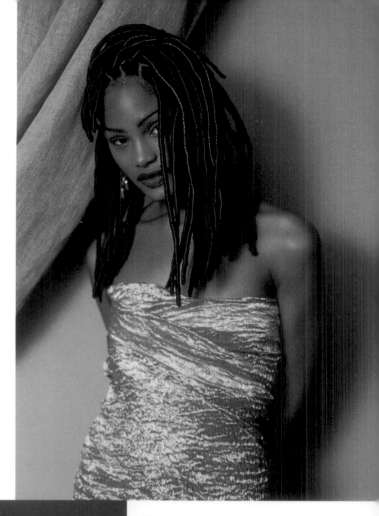

Photograph by John Peden for *Essence*. Courtesy *Essence*

"Silky Dreads — a massive head of individual braids that are placed in from the scalp to the desired length. They are then wrapped individually with Kanekelon hair from the top to the bottom and sealed with heat, giving the braids a silky look. Braid sizes may vary from large to small. Large braids that closely resemble thread wraps can be tied together and arranged high on the head."

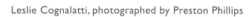

Leslie Cognalatti, photographed by Preston Phillips

"Thread wrapping was once done with plant fibers. Commercial thread now makes color variations possible. Other fibers are also being used, such as yarn, synthetic hair, beaded thread, metallic thread, and embroidery thread."

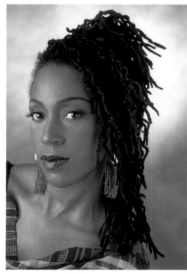

Annu Prestonia, photographed by Yusuf Rashad

"Here is 'Little Egypt' — locks that are groomed, crimped, and colored crimson red and sun-sparkled brown. For those who can't wait the years it takes to grow this style, extensions called 'Cosmic Locks' are available."

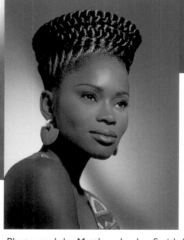

Photograph by Matthew Jordan-Smith for *Essence*. Courtesy *Essence*

"This is the Nefertiti, a style that emulates a famous former queen of Egypt. Four Goddess braids make this one of our all-time most requested braid styles."

Clients

Tempest Bledsoe

Angela Davis

Queen Latifah

Joie Lee

Spike Lee

Oprah Winfrey

Iman

Beverly Peele

Angela Bassett

Beatrice Berry

M-Hotep

Gary Byrd

Germaine Ellis

Jennifer Ivy

Annabelle Baptiste

Wynetta Johnson

Sandy Lewis

Terry McMillan

Imani Monroe

Stephanie Penceal

Jackie Sapp

Stevie Wonder

Alfre Woodard

Diane Worley

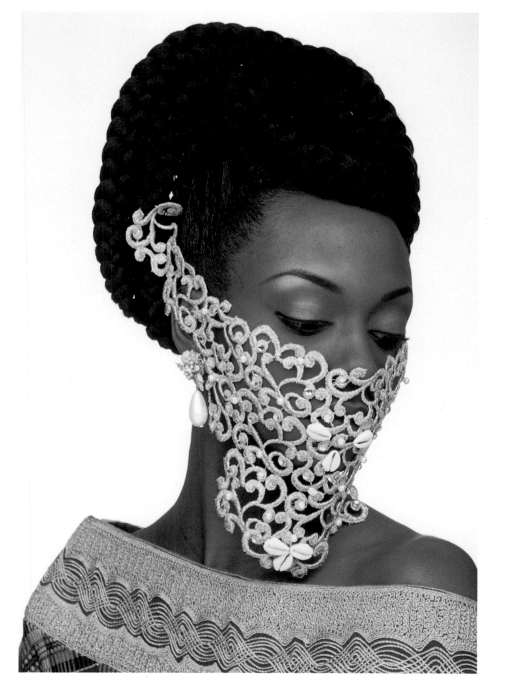

Tammy Grimes, with hair styled by Ruth Sinclair of Khamit Kinks, Atlanta, photographed by Darryl Lane

"The Veiled Goddess Collection — hairstyles and veils that were created for brides. The hair is styled with sculptured Goddess braids. Some are braided off the head and pinned on later. The veil is made of embroidered lace accentuated with pearls, cowrie shells, and rhinestones."

DIDIER MALIGE

Flexibility and the Unexpected

Radical opinions lurk just beneath Didier Malige's mild exterior. For example, he waxes nostalgic about punk hair, a moment in fashion history most of us would rather forget. "That movement was a revelation – the punks invented a whole new way of doing hair. They used colors no one had ever seen before. Hair was as elaborate as in the 18th century, except they were doing it themselves." And what other outré hair statements excite Malige's imagination? "White people with dreadlocks. There's a guy at Ralph Lauren who wears them with pin-striped suits." While Malige reveres extravagant artifice, he also has a weakness for Eve-in-the-Garden-of-Eden naturalness. "I'm in awe of any guy or girl who has very long, virgin, untouched hair," he confesses. "Especially if it's red. I admire any kind of extreme determination with hair."

Determination is clearly one of Malige's own great qualities. It has carried him on a direct course from working as an obscure Parisian salon apprentice to one of the world's top studio stylists. "In France, when you choose a profession as a young person, you are in it for life. It's not like in America, where one day you're a hair-dresser, the next day you're a disk jockey, and after that you sell real estate." He began practicing his craft at 15, when he apprenticed for three years at the celebrated Carita salon, where Jeanne Moreau picked up her hair-pieces and Otto Preminger sent Jean Seberg for her Joan of Arc crop. (The proprietresses, Rosy and Maria Carita, were also the first *grands coiffeurs*.) "For me Carita was the best salon in Paris," he says. "Alexandre's clients were aristocrats and film stars. Carita attracted more intellectual types, especially up-and-coming film stars" – such as Catherine Deneuve, whose hair he vividly recalls drying. He began by passing hairpins, and after that, "I was allowed to touch hair. Then maybe they'd let me place two or three curlers at the back of the neck." The Carita stylist who "most marked" his life was Laurent Gaudefroy. "I don't think anyone works like him any-more. He did 40 clients a day." A master of the chignon, "he made the most amazing forms with hair and taught

Kirsty Hume, photographed by Patrick Demarchelier for *Harper's Bazaar*. Courtesy *Harper's Bazaar* © Hearst Magazines Division

"It takes forever to get dead-straight hair to look this perfect. To achieve the smoothness, I saturated the hair with liquid silicone which gives control and sheen, but is never heavy or greasy."

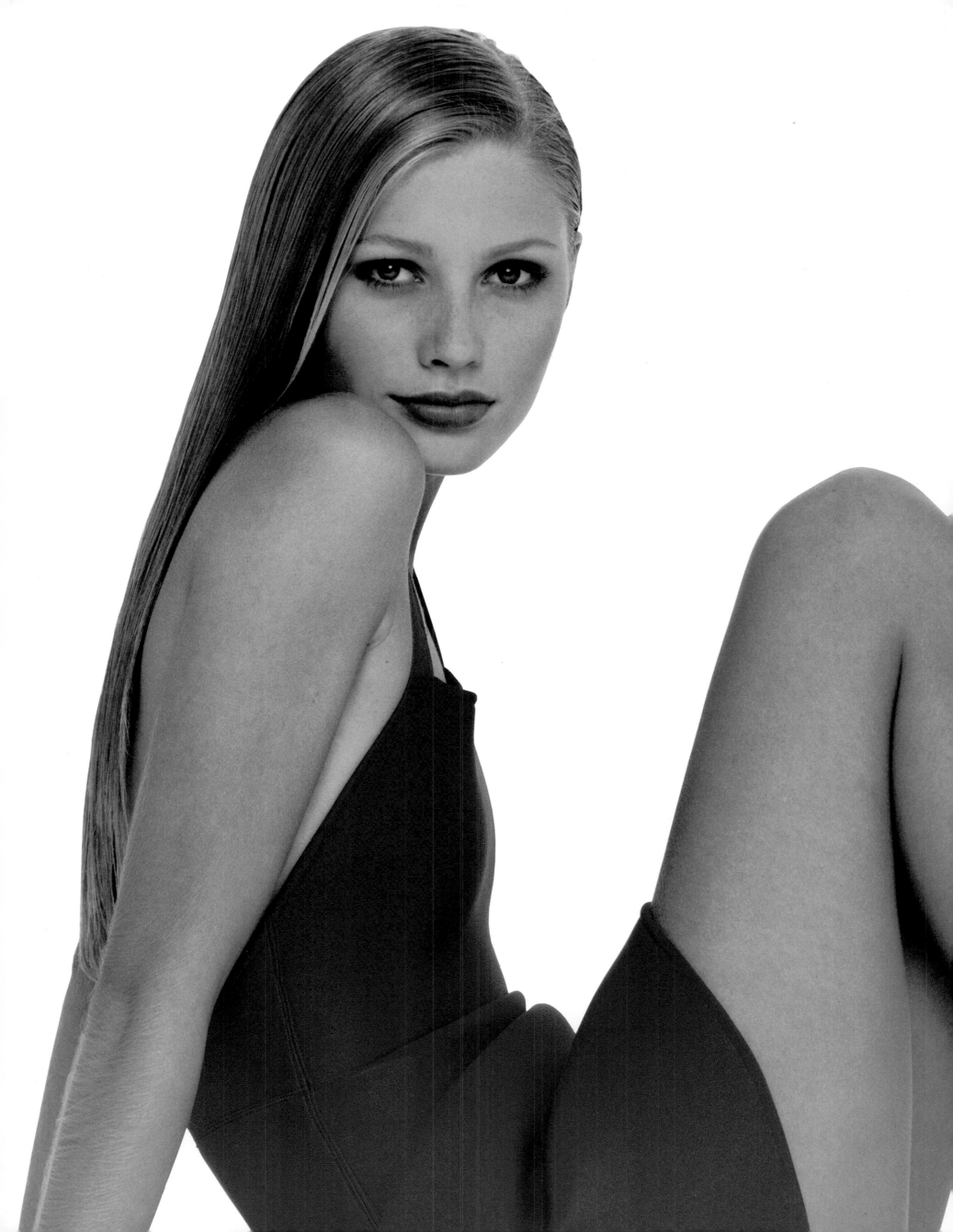

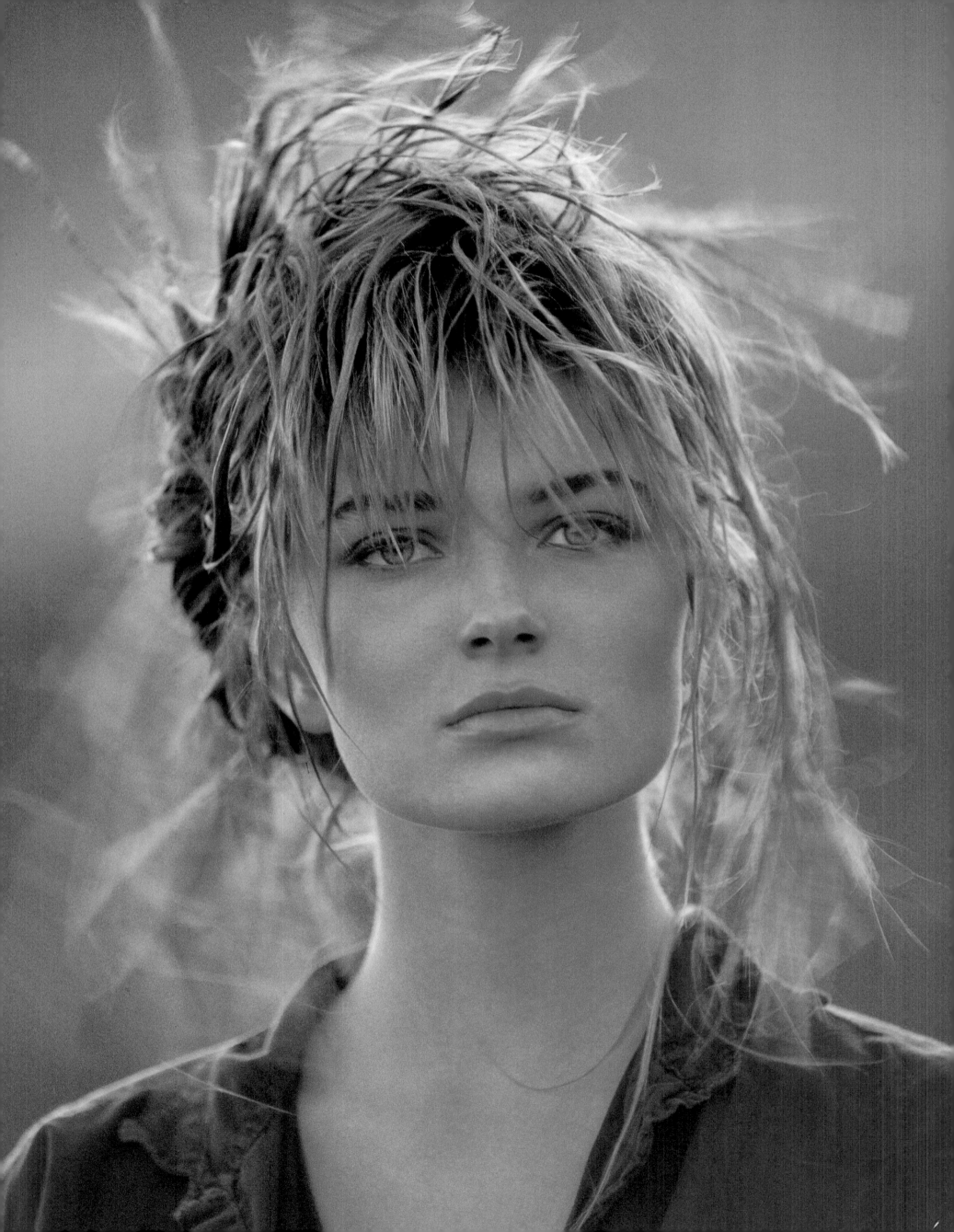

Hairstory

STYLIST: *Didier Malige*
SALON ADDRESS: *The Frederic Fekkai Beauty Center,*
Bergdorf Goodman, 754 Fifth Avenue, New York City
PLACE OF BIRTH: *Neuilly, France*
FIRST JOB: *Age 12, picking raspberries*
TRADEMARKS: *Unpredictability; Gentle manner; No private clients;*
Discipline; All or nothing devotion to his work; Radical opinions

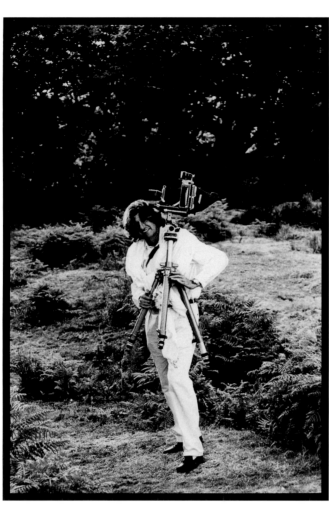

Didier Malige, photographed by Arthur Elgort

me discipline" – a lesson Malige eagerly absorbed, in spite of his $50-a-month pittance. At night he attended school, where he studied everything from back combing to shampoo chemistry.

Malige next moved to the Jean Louis David salon. His boss, the legendary Jean Louis, sent him out to do "a new kind of work that had just begun in the late 60s" – hairstyling for magazine fashion shoots. Though Jean Louis David alone received credit for the hairstyles in the pictures taken by Helmut Newton, Bob Richardson, and Guy Bourdin for French *Vogue*, *Elle*, and *Marie Claire*, Malige was more than delighted. "It was a time when everyone wanted to be either a fashion photographer or a hairdresser. Vidal Sassoon was a big influence on the profession. He made the hairdresser into a very fashionable person." Eventually Jean Louis suggested that Malige curtail the studio work and return to the salon as manager. Malige instead boldly decided to work exclusively as an editorial hairstylist, without any salon affiliation – at that time an arrangement "virtually unheard-of."

As many of the younger European photographers with whom he had previously collaborated – Alex Chatelaine, Patrick Demarchelier – had already migrated to America, Malige decided in 1974 to follow in their wake. "You could make as much in a day in New York as you did in a week in Paris," he says. Nevertheless,

he claims he was at first "not very good at doing American-type hair. Hair was big, more 'done.' In France, hair had already been loosened up, deconstructed." He shrewdly turned his weakness into a strength by working for *Glamour* and *Mademoiselle*, magazines whose younger outlooks allowed him "more freedom with hair." Ads (a much bigger source of revenue than magazines) for Clairol and Celanese quickly came his way. Malige's calling card was "not doing what people expected." He has since added to that trait a reputation for flexibility. "People know I can be pushed into extravagance, but that I can be classic too," he says.

Malige has participated in some of the most visible ad campaigns ever mounted. In conjunction with photographer Bruce Weber, he has styled hair for 12 years' worth of Ralph Lauren ads as well as the occasional Calvin Klein spread. Other accounts include TSE Cashmere – with photographer Patrick Demarchelier – the Gap, and Valentino. (Assignments come through the photographer, rather than directly from the advertiser.) Of all the models he's worked with, he most admires Christy Turlington. "She is disciplined, and good to travel with." He respects Linda Evangelista for her fearless, chameleon-like ability to change her look. And he fondly recalls doing Brooke Shields' hair for an *Elle* cover when the barely adolescent model had just

Paulina Porizkova, photographed by Hans Feurer for American *Vogue*. Courtesy American *Vogue* ©The Condé Nast Publications Inc.

"This was shot for a Vogue beauty story, but it was too much for them and so was never published. I dreadlocked the hair
with a variety of products, which gave it a structural volume much like the real thing."

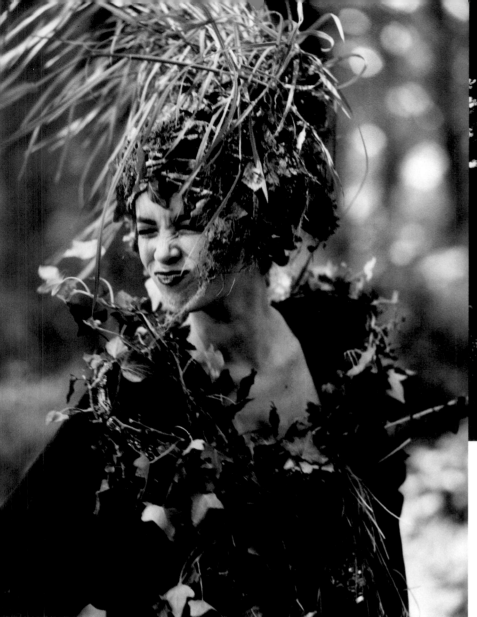

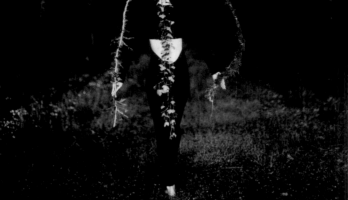

Linda Speering, photographed by Bruce Weber for Karl Lagerfeld

"These pictures were all taken on location at an ancient castle in Brittany, France, and the surroundings inspired the styling of both the shoot and the hair. It was such a mystical, magical place. Karl Lagerfeld gave us total freedom, which was wonderful and quite unusual, but also there was fantastic chemistry among the team gathered for this shoot. We were out in the forest, where, of course, there were branches, tall grasses, and leaves everywhere, and we just started picking them up and putting them on the model. The surroundings made us all a little crazy, and soon there was moss all over the dresses and this great Dutch model was balancing logs on her head. It was wonderful, like a fairy tale and very natural."

finished the movie *Pretty Baby*. "She was very cute – she brought a whole group of her school friends to the studio with her," he says. Malige appreciates the luxury he has of styling only beautiful women's hair. "No matter what you do to them, they cannot look ugly." But his natural reserve inhibits him from forming close friendships with models. "I always keep some distance," he says. "I don't get involved in their lives." On the whole, Malige prefers styling to cutting, which he is more likely to do for men or boys. One of his great passions, in fact, is cutting children's hair. "The proportions of a kid's head are fantastic. The skull is much more exaggerated, the head much rounder, and the forehead higher. I love to make giant cowlicks."

Not surprisingly, Malige has no regrets about renouncing salon work. "I wouldn't be good in a salon. There's a lot more pressure – that's why I don't like runway work either – and you always have to be in a good mood. Clients come expecting to have fun, and you do have to listen to their problems. You really should be in the salon five days a week, so it's difficult to do studio work at the same time." (For business reasons, his magazine credits read "Didier Malige for Frederic Fekkai," even though he

cannot be booked there for appointments; he does, however, help train the stylists.)

His line of work, he wants it known, has its down sides. "You're away from home a lot, traveling to France and Italy," explains Malige, who wouldn't mind more time at his house in the Hamptons. "Your family has to be secondary to your profession. You can't have a nine-to-five lifestyle." If these caveats simply make Malige's work sound more glamorous, he has plenty more cautionary advice to offer the would-be studio stylist. "I know a lot of young people want to do this kind of work. You can make a lot of money. But you cannot be any good at 21 or 22 because you have to mature, and be willing to work as part of a team. A bad attitude is as destructive in this profession as disease and drugs. You can't be brutal, trying to force your point of view on others." In fact, he warns, more often than not the stylist has to subordinate his ego to the photographer's vision. "After all, you're not the boss. Helmut Newton always says, 'There's only one star here, and it's me.' If he doesn't like the hair, he won't take the picture. I happen to like having photographers as directors." Cooperation with a good photographer, he emphasizes, is of the

Linda Evangelista, photographed by Bruce Weber for Gianni Versace Couture

"To shoot the Versace Couture collection, photographer Bruce Weber had us all go to his camp in New York State's Adirondack Mountains. Someone had found the bird's nest, which we all admired. I had the bird models already and thought I'd use both props on top of Linda's classic chignon."

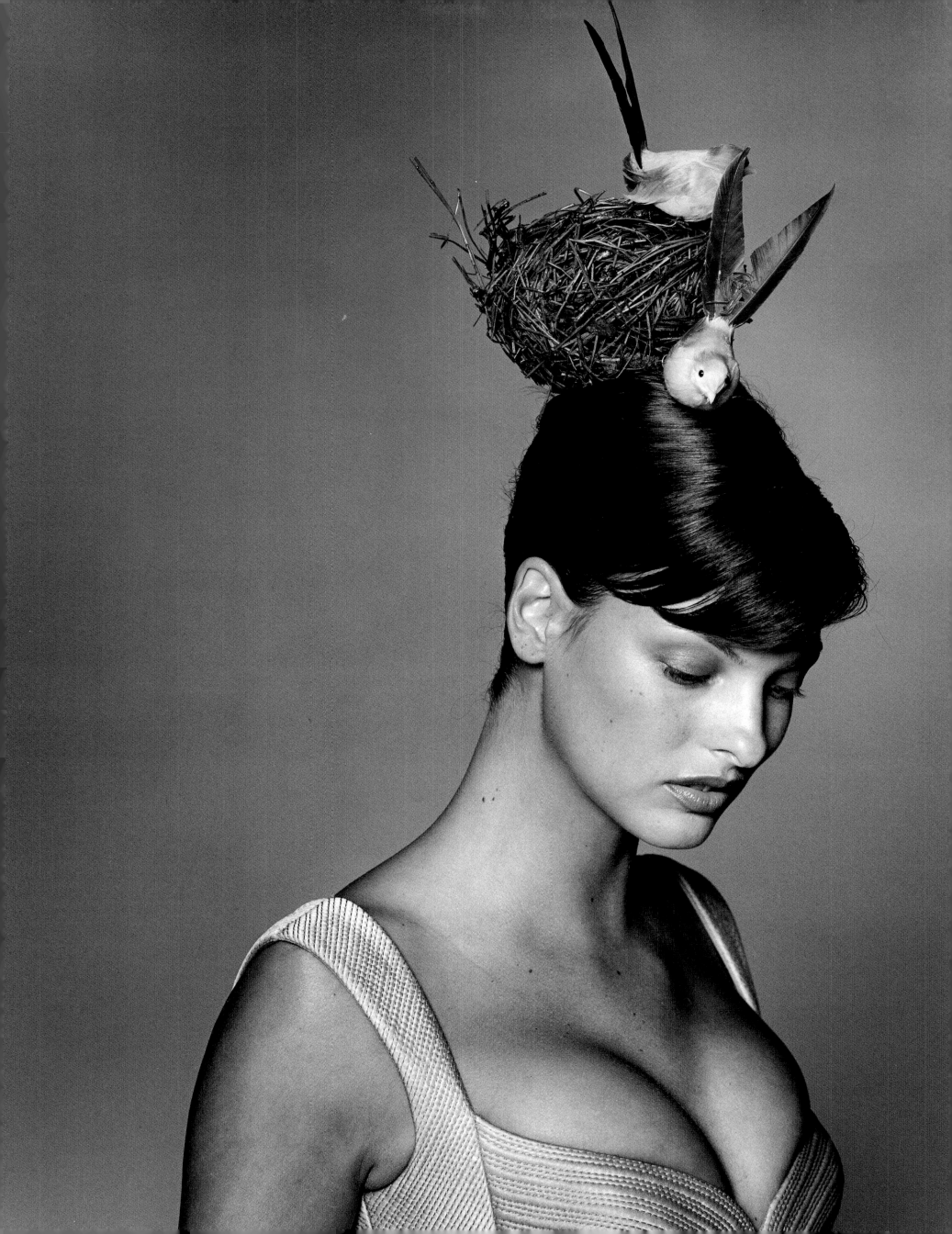

Uma Thurman and Mona, photographed by Sheila Metzner for British *Vogue*. Courtesy British *Vogue* ©The Condé Nast Publications Ltd.

"Uma Thurman was still a teenager at this time, and very lively. She was modeling on her days off from school. On a separate occasion, I had been on a shoot in Mexico with Uma, near Tijuana, and we were nearly attacked by a pack of wild dogs. It ended well, but it was a frightening experience. The dog mask you see Uma wearing on her head in these images is a reference to that experience.

"The shoot itself took place in Barry Friedman's gallery on Madison Avenue in New York City. I was inspired by the grace and beauty of the architecture and the stunning pre-Raphaelite paintings that he was exhibiting at the time. Also, the photographer, Sheila Metzner, was a close friend of Uma's mother, so a few different strands came together on this project.

"Mona's hair was long and extremely curly, but I wound it up in this way to make her look like a little animal. All around us was fantasy . . . in the paintings, in the clothes, and so also, I hope, in the hair."

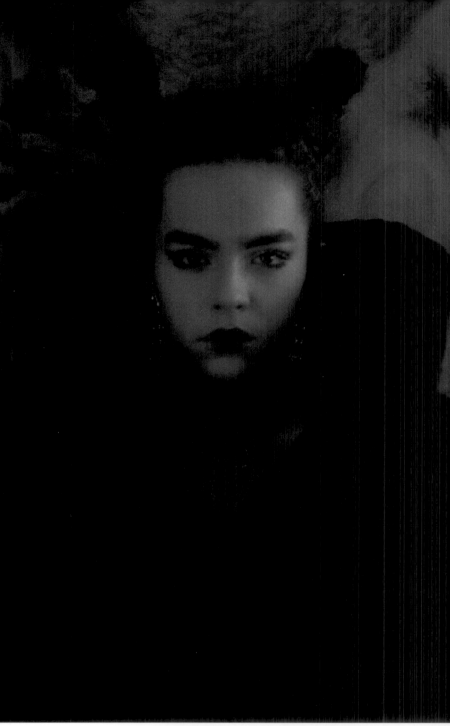

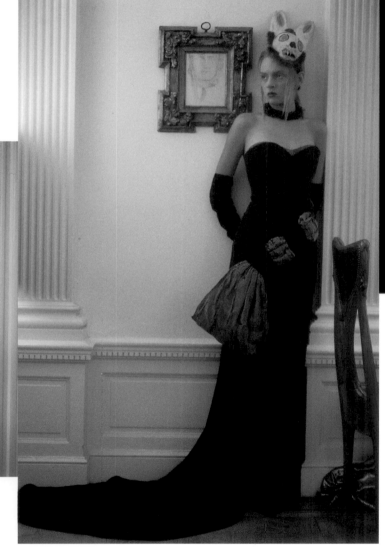

Isabelle Pasco, photographed by Lord Snowdon for British *Vogue*. Courtesy British *Vogue* ©The Condé Nast Publications Ltd.

"Lord Snowdon and I worked together on this shoot for Chanel's winter couture collection. Snowdon wanted to shoot against this richly painted backdrop of a formal garden, and I have always loved topiaries, which became my inspiration for the hair."

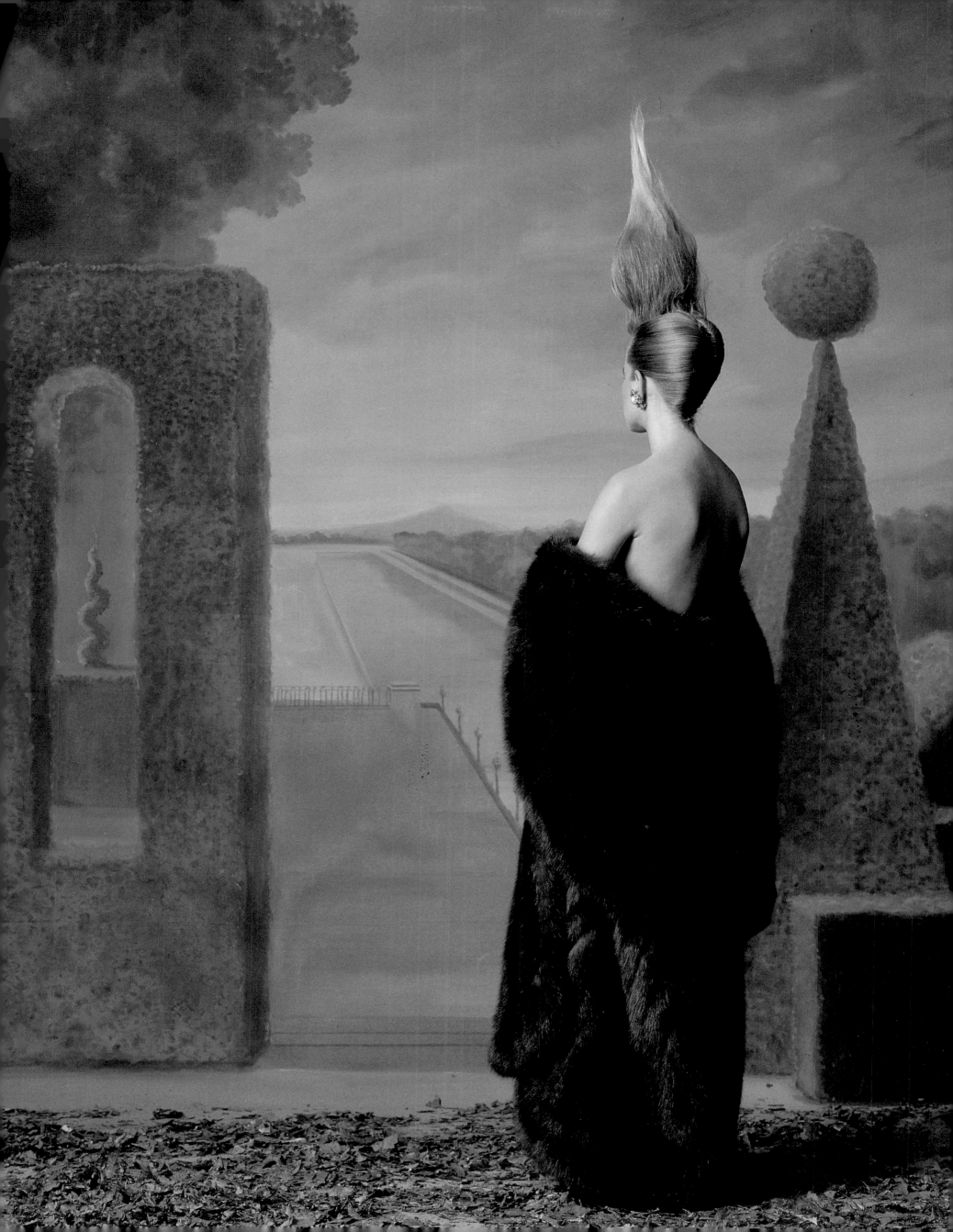

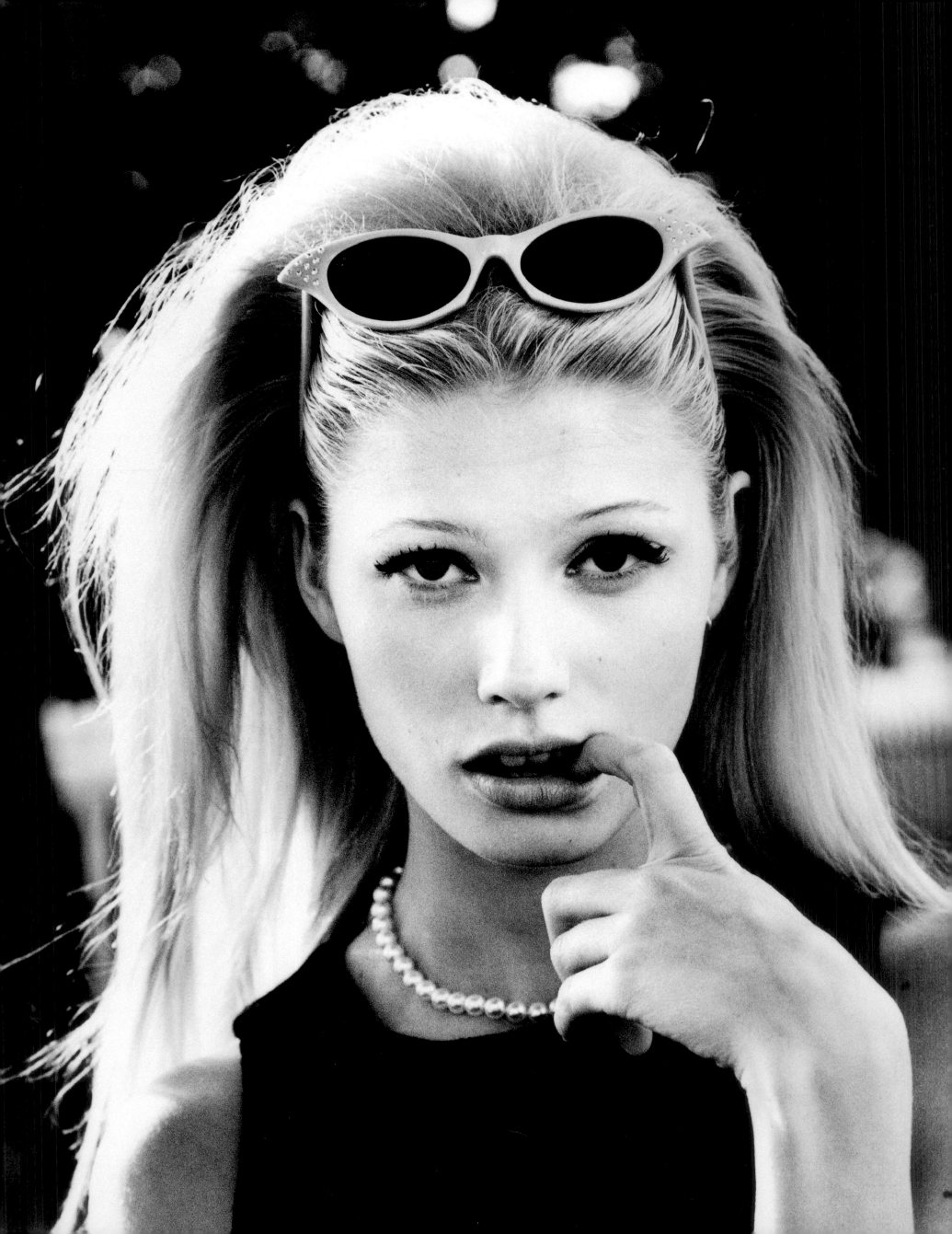

"This photograph was a tribute, of sorts, to the work of Diane Arbus: the idea of a lost soul in a public place. I curled Kate Moss' hair with a tiny 'Marcel' curling iron, and then teased the hair out. The semi-transparent dress makes this picture feel very late 1960s to me."

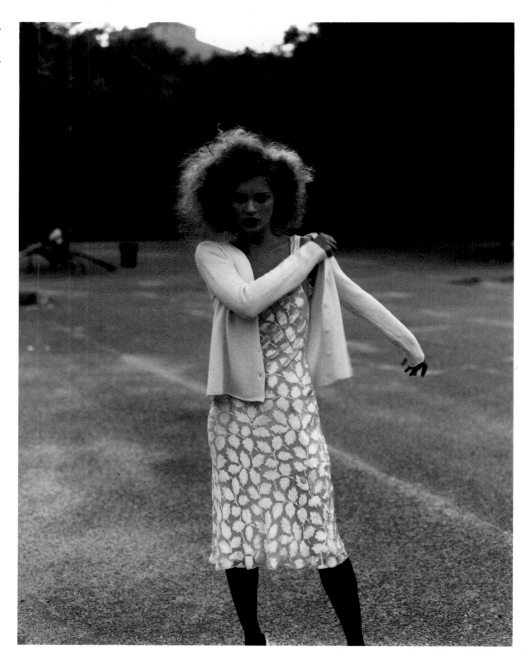

utmost importance, because in the end "it is he who makes you successful. Who would notice your work without the pictures?"

Though the closest Malige gets to the heads of ordinary people is the occasional on-the-job trim of a fashion editor, he has an abundance of helpful pointers from which the average woman can profit. If you don't have access to, or cannot afford, a great stylist, he recommends a conservative haircut. "Women often try too hard, or want to be too trendy," he says. He proposes a Louise Brooks-type bob with bangs as one look that is "never out of fashion." But he cautions against any length that settles between the chin and the shoulders. "It has to hit in the right place – at the jawline or above – otherwise you look ten years older." As much as aging coifs, he dislikes (except on the most gorgeous models) severely asymmetric styles and those "that make women look like transvestites" – that is, big hair that resembles a wig. "Only Dolly Parton can get away with that." Eccentricity is acceptable, as long as a woman is absolutely confi-

dent that it suits her. Excessive perming and overbleaching, he feels, is an epidemic among women in Los Angeles. With their hair "curly on top and floppy on the sides," the women end up "looking like poodles." He has a particular horror of home perming – the trickiest procedure of all do-it-yourself haircare; instead, he encourages the creation of waves with a curling iron – his favorite tool. "I don't know how to do a perfect blow-dry," he admits. "What I *am* good at is hiding my mistakes!" To simulate the "smooth, shiny, luxuriant" appearance of immaculately blown-dry hair, he coats strands with a silicone-based product such as Sebastian Laminates. Mousse is his first choice for thickening hair; gel he deems best on men because, once applied, it doesn't allow for change; and spray, he believes, is the best product "for construction." Finally, he admonishes the fainthearted, "Don't be afraid to cut your hair. Experiment. Find your own style. People recognize and remember you first by your hair."

"We shot this story in London, and were going for a 1960s feel. Although women frequently used hairpieces to create a style like this in the 60s, Kirsty has very long hair so I didn't need one. However, in order to get volume I used a 60s trick ... dry shampoo. I applied it to the roots and then brushed it out."

Likes

CUT:
classic straight hair
chin-length bob with bangs

COLOR:
red
punk multicolors

STYLE:
Caucasians with Rastafarian locks
early 80s experimental hair
waves created with hot irons
fearlessness
traditional styling when access to a top hairdresser is limited

TREATMENT:
mousse
spray
gel
silicone-based hair products for sheen

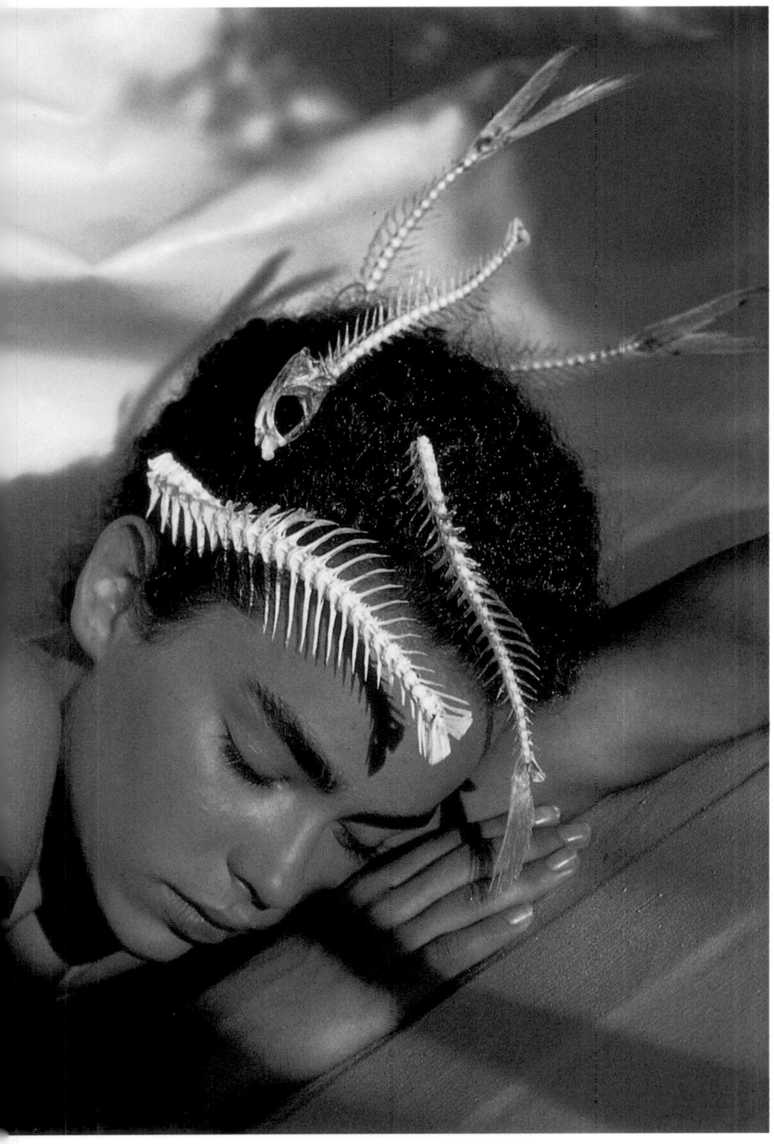

Dislikes

CUT:
hair lengths that hit between the chin and shoulder

COLOR:
overbleaching

STYLE:
home perms
extreme geometric styles that cause gender confusion

Mona, photographed by Alex Chatelaine for British *Vogue*.
Courtesy British *Vogue* ©The Condé Nast Publications Ltd.

"Hairstyling using props from lunch."

Mona, photographed by Alex Chatelaine for British *Vogue*.
Courtesy British *Vogue* ©The Condé Nast Publications Ltd.

"These pictures were the result of perfect teamwork. We shot on a private island in the Caribbean, and everyone's creativity was flowing like crazy. The hair in this image is a hairpiece from the shoulders down."

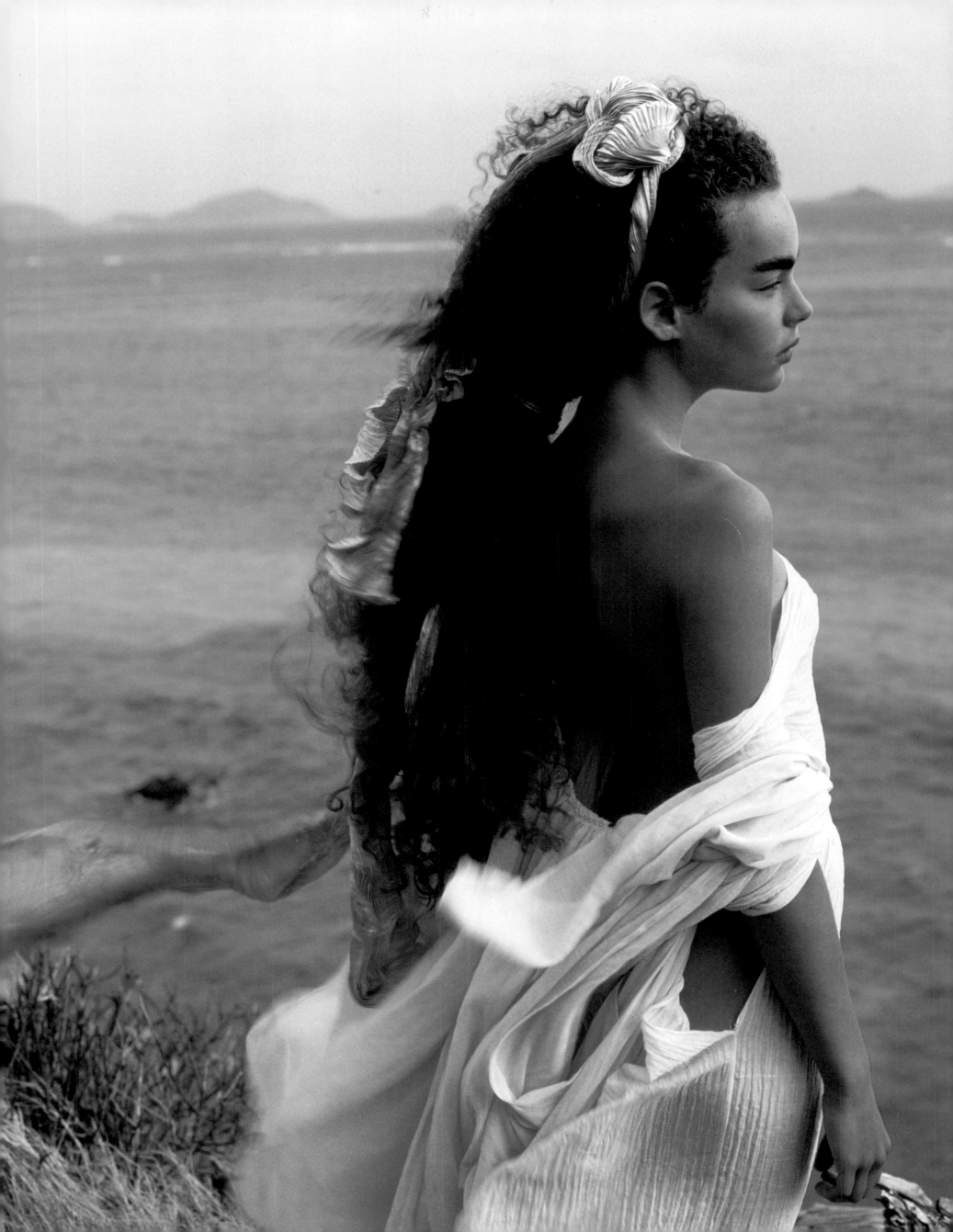

Linda Evangelista, photographed by Bruce Weber for Gianni Versace

"This was part of a campaign for men's clothing for Versace. We thought that Linda Evangelista would look great as a man. The hair is classic Elvis Presley, one of the most timeless men's hairstyles."

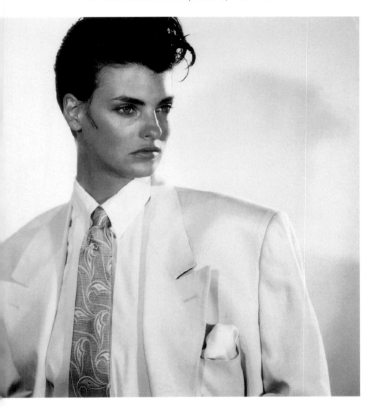

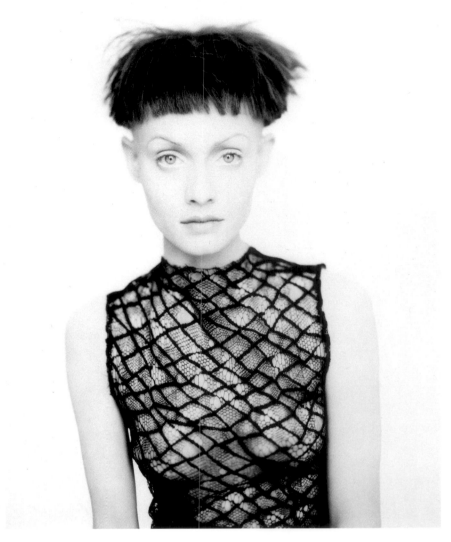

Amber Valetta, photographed by Paolo Roversi for *Harper's Bazaar*. Courtesy *Harper's Bazaar*

"I hid Amber's own hair under a bald cap to give the illusion that her head had been shaved. Then I put a wig on top and cut it into this blunt, futuristic-medieval style."

Do's & Don'ts

Fashion contradicts itself. Therefore:
Don't Worry
Do It
Do Change the Color
Do Cut It
Your hair will always grow back.

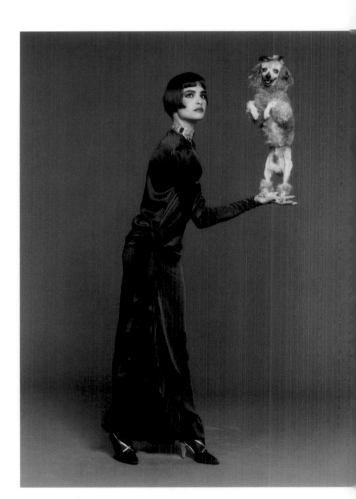

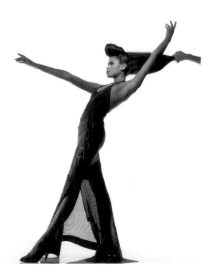

Gail O'Neal, photographed by Patrick Demarchelier for British *Vogue*. Courtesy British *Vogue* ©The Condé Nast Publications Ltd.

"I am always inspired by Spanish women, especially dancers, with their hair combs and graceful, rhythmic hand movements. That is actually my hand holding her hair from outside the frame. I was just holding the hair and photographer Patrick Demarchelier told me to stay where I was."

Talisa Soto, photographed by Bruce Weber for British *Vogue*. Courtesy British *Vogue* ©The Condé Nast Publications Ltd.

"This photograph, shot in Paris, was never published, reportedly because the dog was a boy. I cut the model's hair into a Louise Brooks bob. It always amazes me how this cut comes back again and again, and always looks fresh. For women with straight, not-too-thick hair and that architectural-type face, it is the most timeless style."

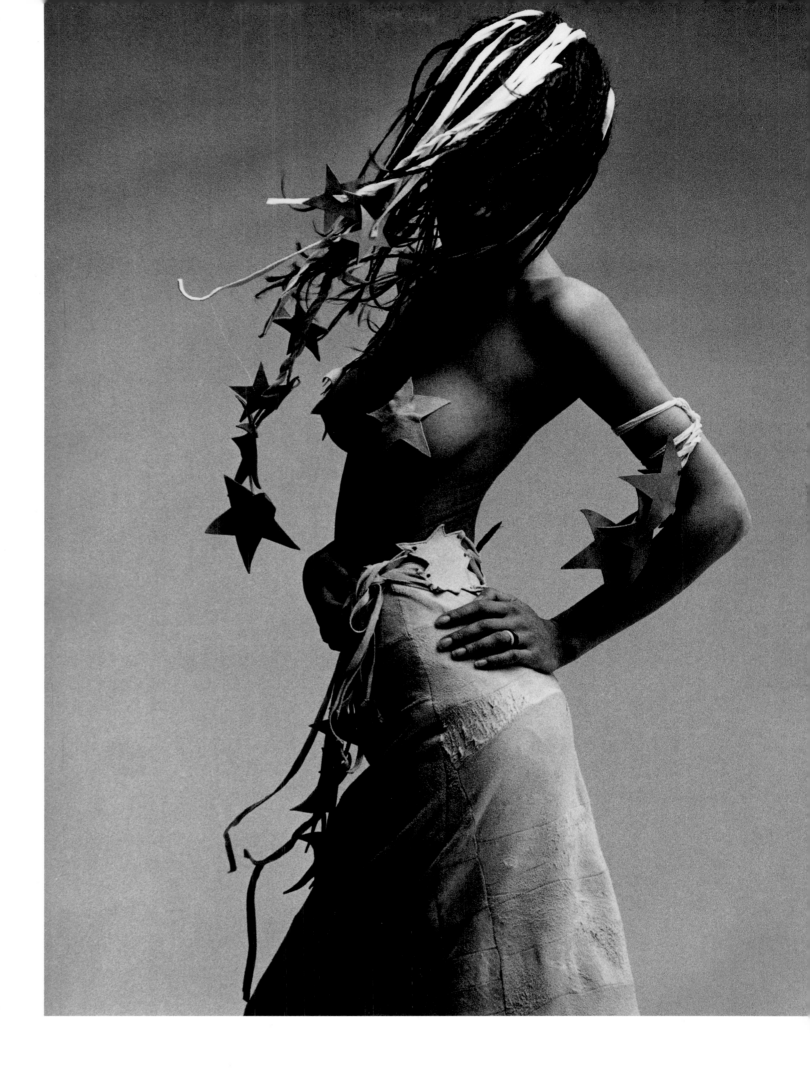

Paula, photographed by Hans Feurer for _Twen_. Courtesy _Twen_

"Shot in Hans Feurer's London studio, this was my first work with Hans and featured a collection of chamois leather clothing by designer Henry Lehr. (Lehr also made his wife's wedding dress out of chamois.) Hans and I spent hours and hours braiding the model's hair the night before the shoot. She had to sleep with the braids, and I had nightmares all night, envisioning each and every braid unravelling."

Cecilla Chancellor, photographed by Hans Feurer for British *Vogue*.
Courtesy British *Vogue* ©The Condé Nast Publications Ltd.

"Here Cecilia appears as if she were in a painting by John Singer Sargent."

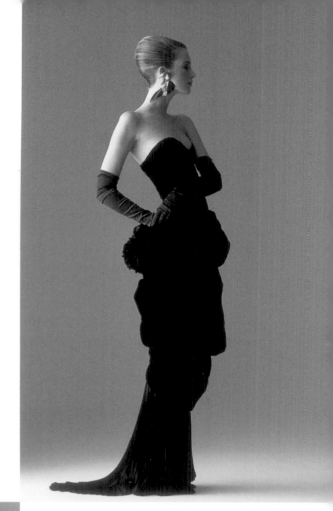

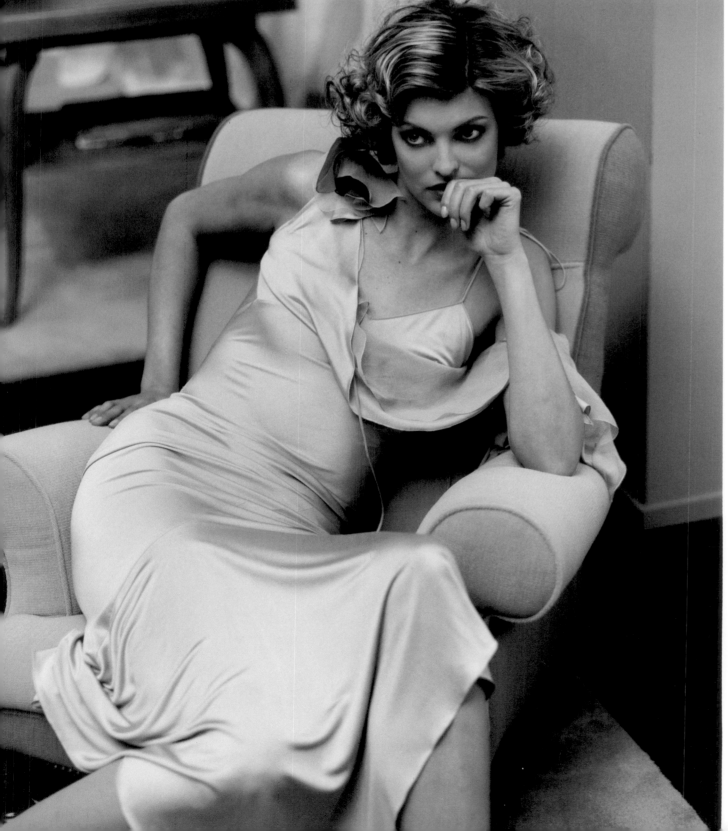

Linda Evangelista, photographed by Steven Meisel for American *Vogue*.
Courtesy American *Vogue* ©The Condé Nast Publications Inc.

"This story was shot at Aero Studios, in New York, where their wonderful furniture and John Galliano's utterly feminine dresses combined to create this very 1940s style. Linda's hair is naturally straight, but I used a curling iron."

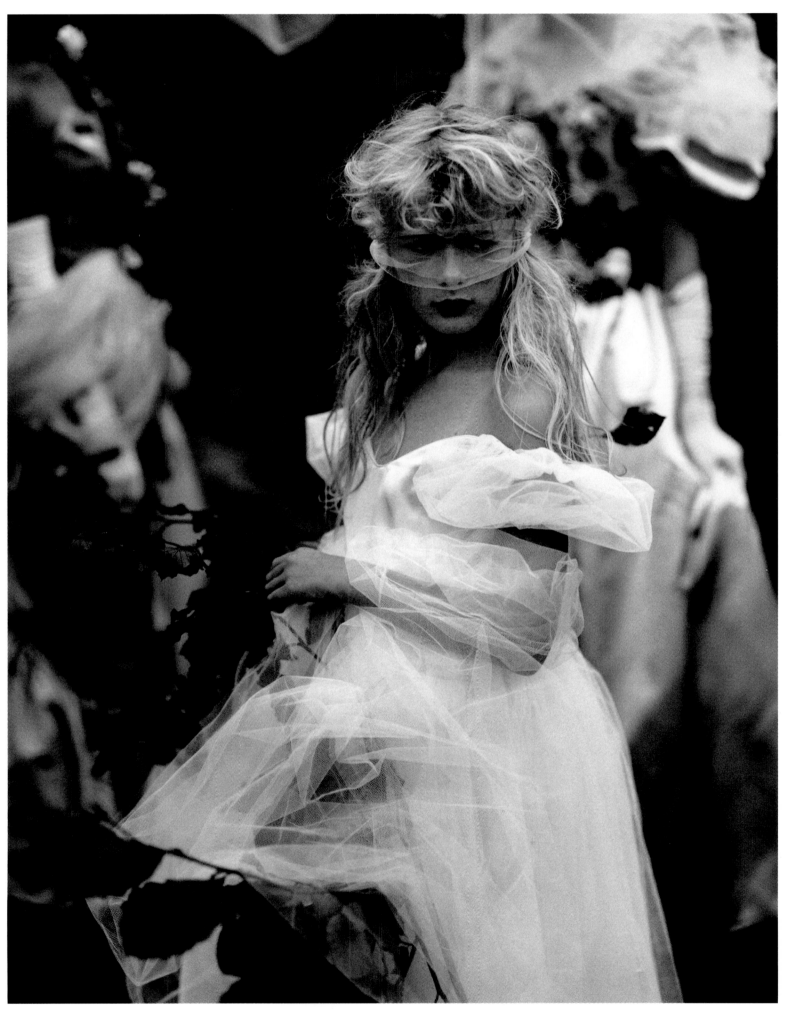

Photograph by Bruce Weber for British *Vogue*. Courtesy British *Vogue* ©The Condé Nast Publications Ltd.

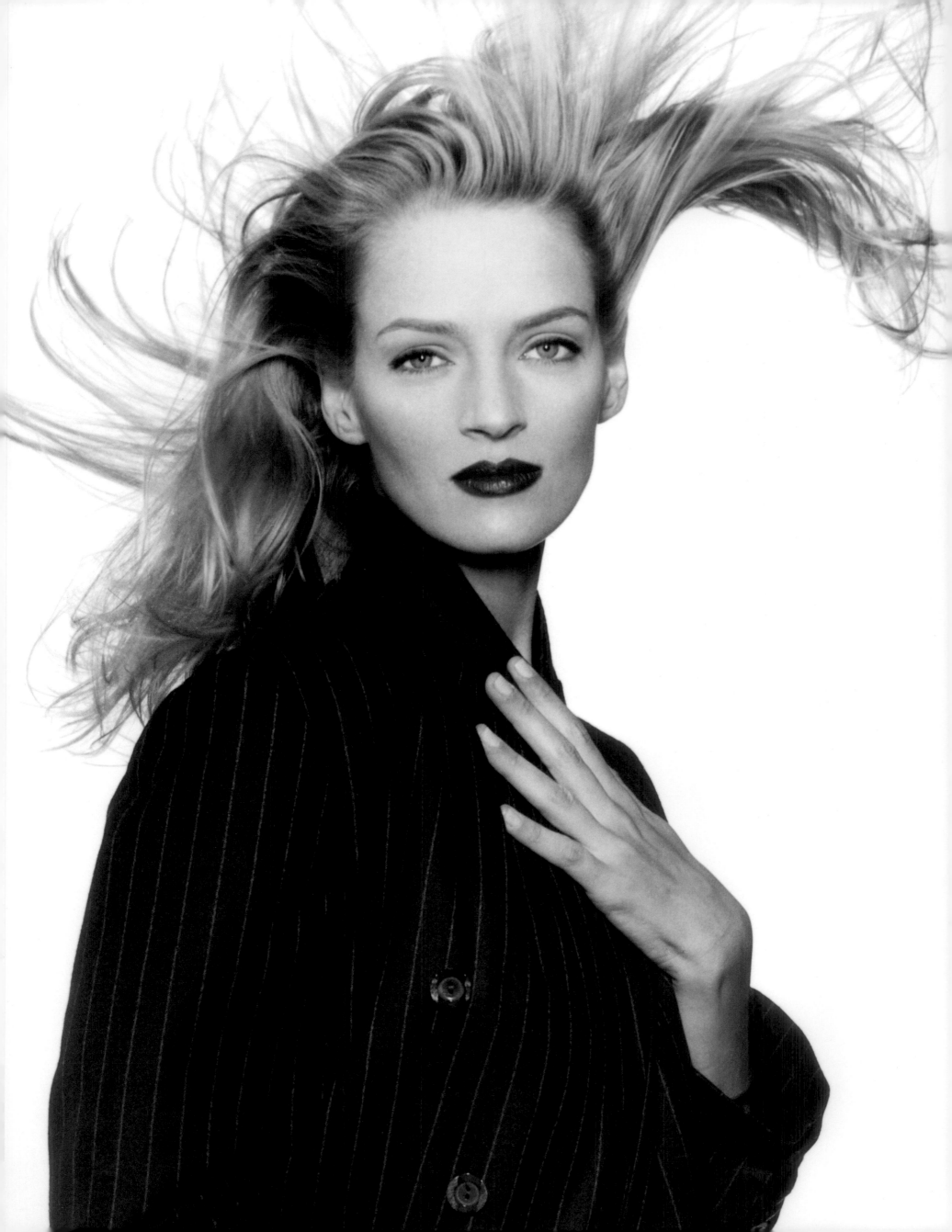

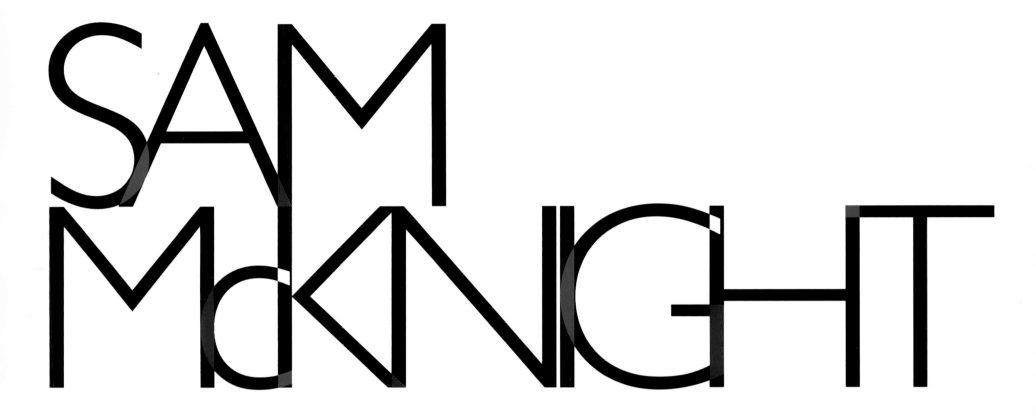

SAM McKNIGHT

Approachable Glamour

Sam McKnight, session stylist, is such a celebrity in the UK that reporters routinely ferret out his parents in a remote hamlet in Scotland for interviews. "It's crazy," says McKnight, a lanky man with close-cropped hair, a goatee, and eyebrows that shoot skyward like a conductor's batons. Once, journalists came to see his mother, she made them tea, and then the paper published a story headlined "He Doesn't Even Cut His Own Mother's Hair!" Of course, the article explained in smaller print that the peripatetic McKnight – who these days is more likely to be found on a plane than in either his London or New York apartment – is rarely near home anymore, and that Mrs. McKnight is very happy indeed to patronize her local beautician.

So what is the reason for this intense public scrutiny? McKnight offers two explanations. First, he has recently launched, via a hugely visible ad campaign, a line of eight top-selling hairstyling products bearing his name, which is stocked throughout the kingdom in the ubiquitous chain drugstore Boots. Second, and more to the point, McKnight has been, for the last five years, the personal hairdresser for Her Royal Highness, The Princess of Wales, whose locks are even more closely watched – and criticized – than Hillary Rodham Clinton's. The buzz generated by this royal client/stylist relationship reached a roaring crescendo in February 1995 when McKnight dared to slick back the Princess's golden curls for her appearance in New York at the Council of Fashion Designers of America's awards ceremony. For some members of the British press, nothing so drastic had been perpetrated on an aristocrat's head since Marie Antoinette's came tumbling off the chopping block. More sophisticated observers applauded the transformation from patrician matron to chic, sleek goddess. Anything else there is to know about his tonsorial connection to the Princess of Wales is a better-kept secret than most goings-on at Buckingham Palace. McKnight assumes an air of impenetrable detachment if any further questions are posed. Not even a "no comment" issues from his tightly sealed lips.

Uma Thurman, photographed by Marc Hispard for French *Vogue*. Courtesy French *Vogue*

"Uma's drop-dead glam. Lifted and separated with Big Mousse."

Her Royal Highness, The Princess of Wales, clearly must appreciate McKnight's discretion, a rarity in a notoriously loose-tongued profession. But, as every supermodel well knows, an acute sense of privacy is just one of McKnight's many commendable qualities. He is renowned as a studio stylist who cares as much about enhancing a woman's self-esteem as he does about his art. "I like it when the women feel good – when I can make them feel glamorous and beautiful. I'm not into making them look ugly. Who likes a scary woman? A woman should look approachable. I hate it when people make women look like drag queens." His genuine empathy for models has not only made them his close friends, it has also made their careers. During a whitewater rafting shoot in Utah for British *Vogue*, he chopped Fabienne's hair boy-short. "We were in the middle of the wilderness, and there were no mirrors. For three days she had no idea what she looked like." But Fabienne's trust in McKnight paid a handsome dividend: she was immediately awarded the Helena Rubinstein contract. Similarly, shearing Beri Smither's hair to her skull changed her from "just another girl" into a "real star." By removing so much hair, he had excavated Smither's amazing face and fantastic bone structure. This does not mean that McKnight is going to come after every aspiring supermodel with a pair of sharp and gleaming scissors. "A lot of women ask me to cut it all off and I won't. I

often know better than they do when the time's right for a drastic change."

In fact, when he's asked to name some of the best hair around, he's inclined to cite longer 'dos. "Cindy Crawford's hair is always fantastic, especially since it's not so big anymore. Uma Thurman's hair is wonderful. Roseanne is great with her straight, simple hair – a real transformation from the stringy perm she started with. Sandra Bernhard always looks good – very groomed, but not over the top." And though Linda Evangelista inclines toward shorter styles, he crowns her "the queen of hair. No matter what she does, it always looks easy, never complicated – even if it's bleached white." Similarly, he finds Naomi Campbell an inspiration for black women, because "she's made her hair so versatile." McKnight, however, has no delusions about the difference between experimental studio coiffures and real-life hair. When called upon to do realistic hair for magazines, runways, or advertisements, he "tries to promote an easy, natural, unconstructed look. He advises mortal women that "it is important not to look like you tried too hard. Which doesn't necessarily mean that no effort is involved. But if you take one hour every morning to do your hair, something is definitely wrong. The biggest mistake I see American women make is doing too much – too much hair, too much bleach, too much color, too much teasing. Also, the

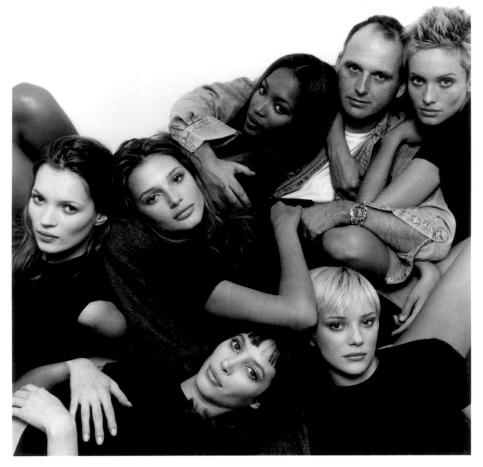

Sam McKnight and friends, photographed by Patrick Demarchelier for British *Marie Claire*. Courtesy British *Marie Claire*

Hairstory

STYLIST: *Sam McKnight*
SALON ADDRESS: *His carry-on flight bag*
PLACE OF BIRTH: *Ayrshire, Scotland*
FIRST JOB: *Age 20, South Molton Street Salon, Scotland, window cleaner*
TRADEMARK: *He can do anyone's hair with congeniality and wit*

Trish Goff and Jaime Richar, photographed by Patrick Demarchelier for *Harper's Bazaar*. Courtesy *Harper's Bazaar* © Hearst Magazines Division

"Super-shiny. Slicked and flipped, with Extreme Gel and Extreme Spray."

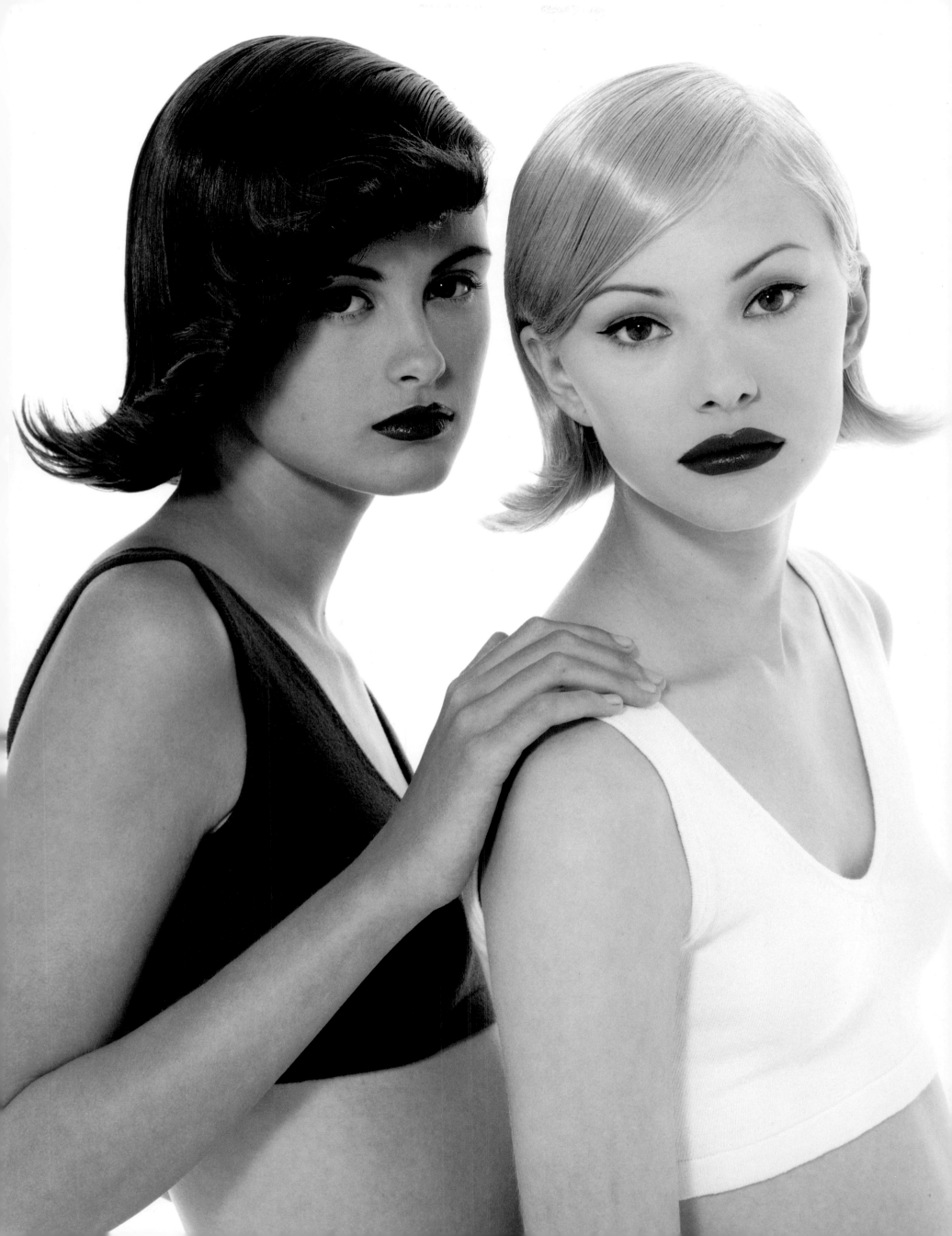

tendency to imitate a style that was featured in *Vogue*. I see my work copied on the street all the time. Just because the hair may have worked on Linda Evangelista, that doesn't necessarily mean it will be right for someone else. You often risk ending up with a caricature of a style." For this reason, he habitually turns away women who call him up offering thousands of dollars to recreate on them a look they admired in a magazine. "It's not what I do," he asserts firmly.

McKnight does advocate that women see their salon hairdresser as often as they can for professional styling, maintenance, and care. "Women in England are more likely to do their hair themselves, with not always terribly good results. It's partly related to this thing English women have about not being too showy or ostentatious. I think American women take better care of their hair in general. There is such good advice in the magazines. And there are so many good products and good salons here."

Though exclusively a session stylist for the last 15 years, McKnight is no stranger to the salon. He entered the profession at 19, through the back door. While studying at a teacher's training college in Scotland to be a French instructor, he came to the realization that he was learning nothing except "how to pass the exams and maybe read the recipes in *Elle* magazine. So I dropped out to try to figure out what to do with my life." Indecisive about his future, he began "driving vans, picking up stock, doing anything" for some friends who owned beauty parlors in Scotland. After observing stylists at work, he thought, half-jokingly at first, "I could do that too – and it turned out I could." Eventually he resolved to "do this the right way," and left for London where he joined the Glemby salon at Elizabeth Arden. In 1977, he relocated to London's fashionable Molton Brown salon, where a "post-hippie" ethos ruled. "Hair had to be completely natural. There were no electric appliances, no setting, and no dryers. The salon was known for shag haircuts, wash-and-wear perms, and for inventing twisting rollers" — conceived as a gentler alternative to electric curlers. All this wariness of sophisticated implements promoted "excellent training in using my hands." McKnight's most memorable experience at Molton Brown was the simultaneous arrival one day of Alana Hamilton, Bianca Jagger, Margaret Trudeau, and Roger Daltry's wife. "For me it was such a moment – all of them there chitchatting away."

Meanwhile, McKnight had been venturing out of the salon, assisting the Molton Brown senior stylists who worked on fashion shows. One day in 1978, a hairdresser scheduled for a

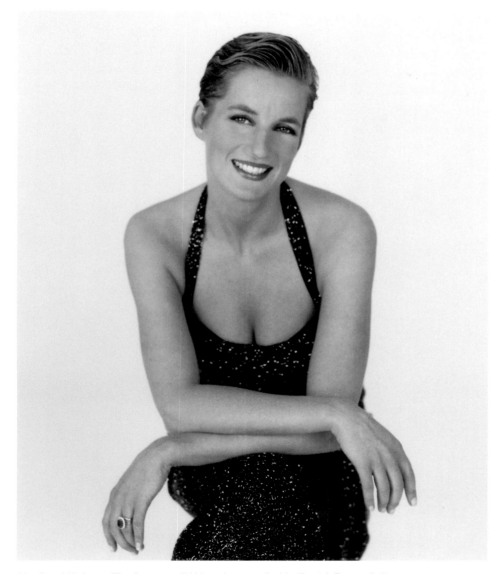

Her Royal Highness, The Princess of Wales, photographed by Patrick Demarchelier

Her Royal Highness, The Princess of Wales, photographed by Patrick Demarchelier

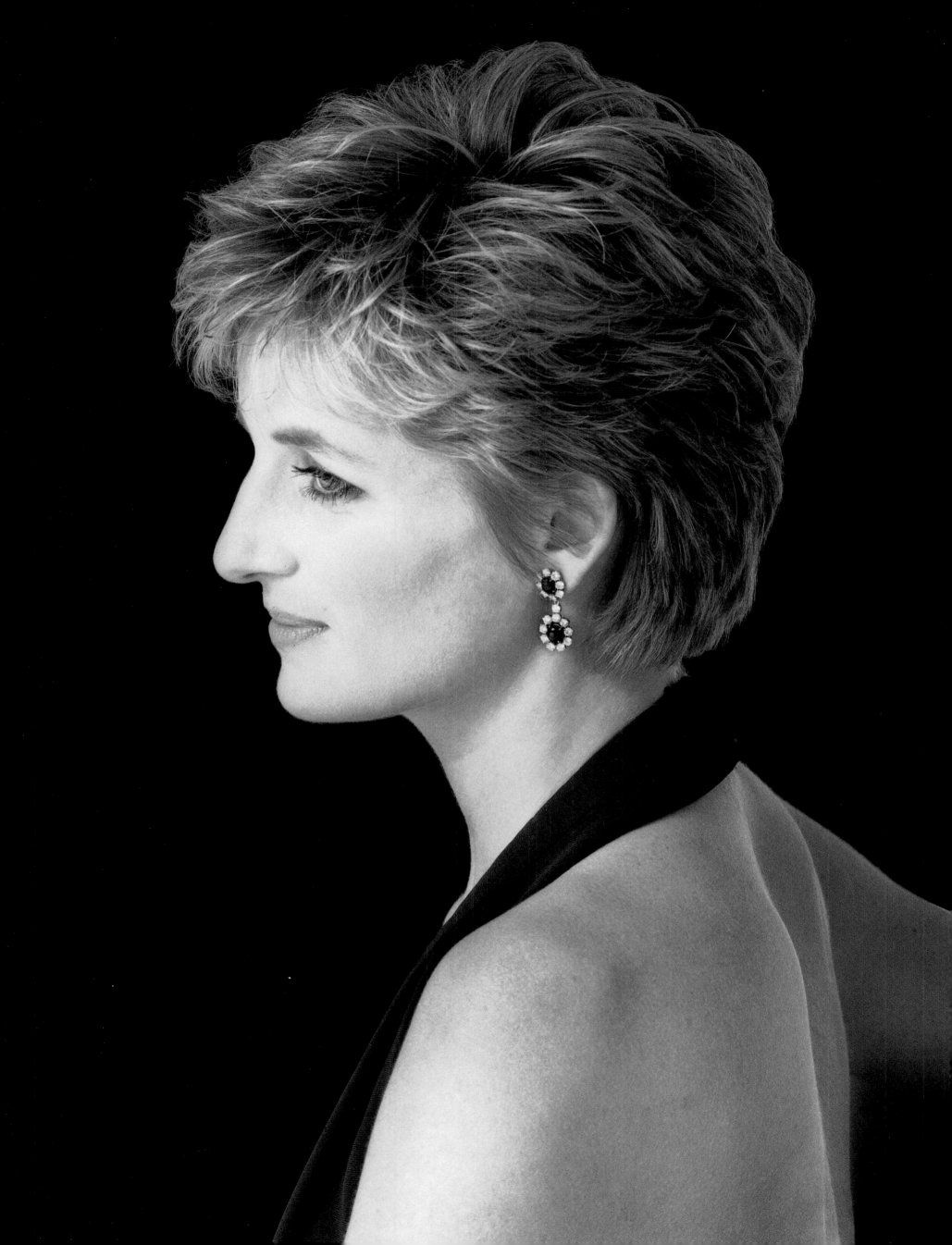

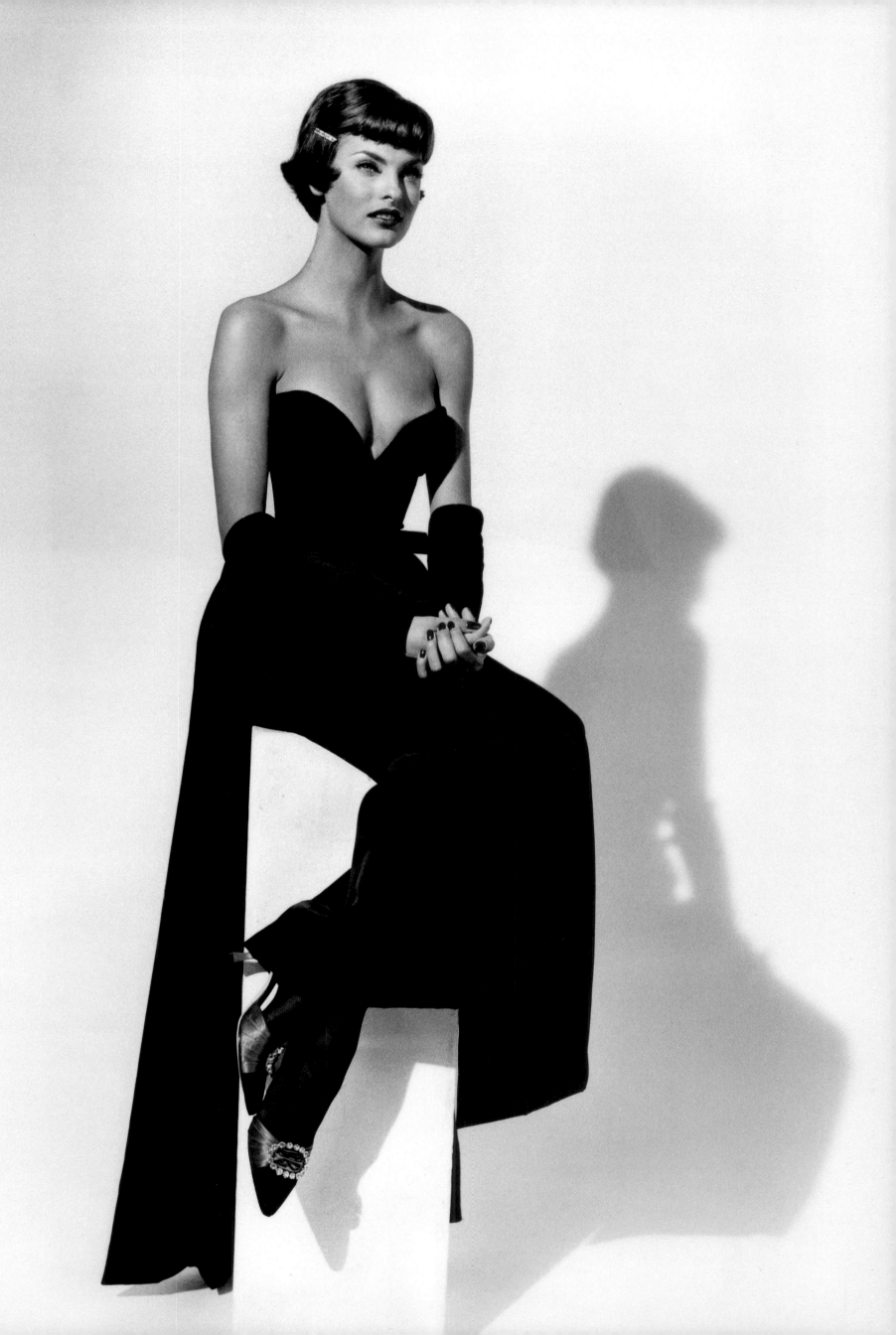

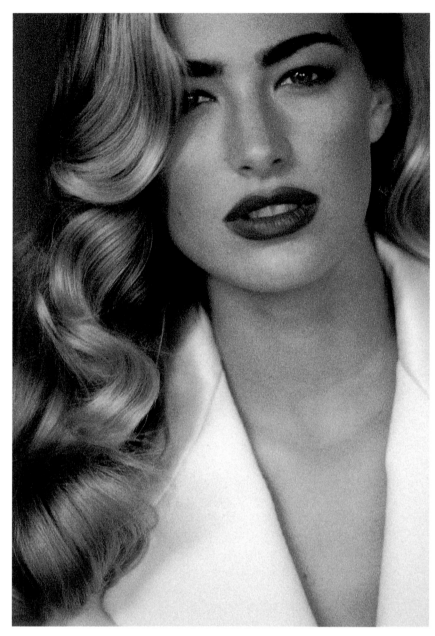

Elaine Irwin, photographed by Sheila Metzner for British *Vogue*.
Courtesy British *Vogue* ©The Condé Nast Publications Ltd.

*"Elaine Irwin's simple, classic Hollywood glamour. A Veronica
Lake for the 90s. Loosely set with Extreme Atomized Gel."*

British *Vogue* shoot with Eric Boman fell ill, and McKnight filled in. Other magazines — most notably the trendy, but now-defunct, *Honey* — began calling, and soon his session assignments overtook his salon work. "It was very difficult to do both," he says. By 1980 he had left Molton Brown to go out on his own as a session stylist. "Today I get all kinds of letters from people who want to be session stylists. When I started, it was a new kind of work. In the early 70s, models did their own hair and makeup. By the late 70s, hairdressers got involved and, soon after, makeup artists — it's always a little harder for a girl to do her hair than her makeup. I think session styling has taken off in a big way because of the whole supermodel phenomenon, the whole explosion of fashion that began in the 80s."

Like other coveted stylists, McKnight worries about the toll that constant jetting across time zones ("I'm home maybe 5% of the year") takes on his body. Typically, during the four weeks of the international ready-to-wear collections, he will do 18 shows in four completely different cities — from Prada in Milan to Vivienne Westwood in Paris, and from Nicole Fahri in London to Anne Klein in New York. Then there are ad campaigns for Ralph Lauren, Revlon, and Versace, among others. He has discovered that losing weight, abstaining from alcohol, and ingesting Chinese herbs to regulate his metabolism have helped keep him fighting trim. Ultimately, the profits from his products and some other McKnight inventions currently under development (the nature of which he won't yet divulge) will allow him to "cut out some of the things I don't want to do." Budding entrepreneur though he may be, McKnight vows he will "continue to do what I do. People like my work because I can do any kind of hair. But I'd also like to think they choose me for my personality too." In his heart, though, McKnight still remains the son of the miner and the grocery clerk from Ayr. "I haven't changed at all," he insists. "Only my accent has!"

Linda Evangelista, photographed by Patrick Demarchelier for British *Vogue*. Courtesy British *Vogue* ©The Condé Nast Publications Ltd.

"Quintessential Evangelista."

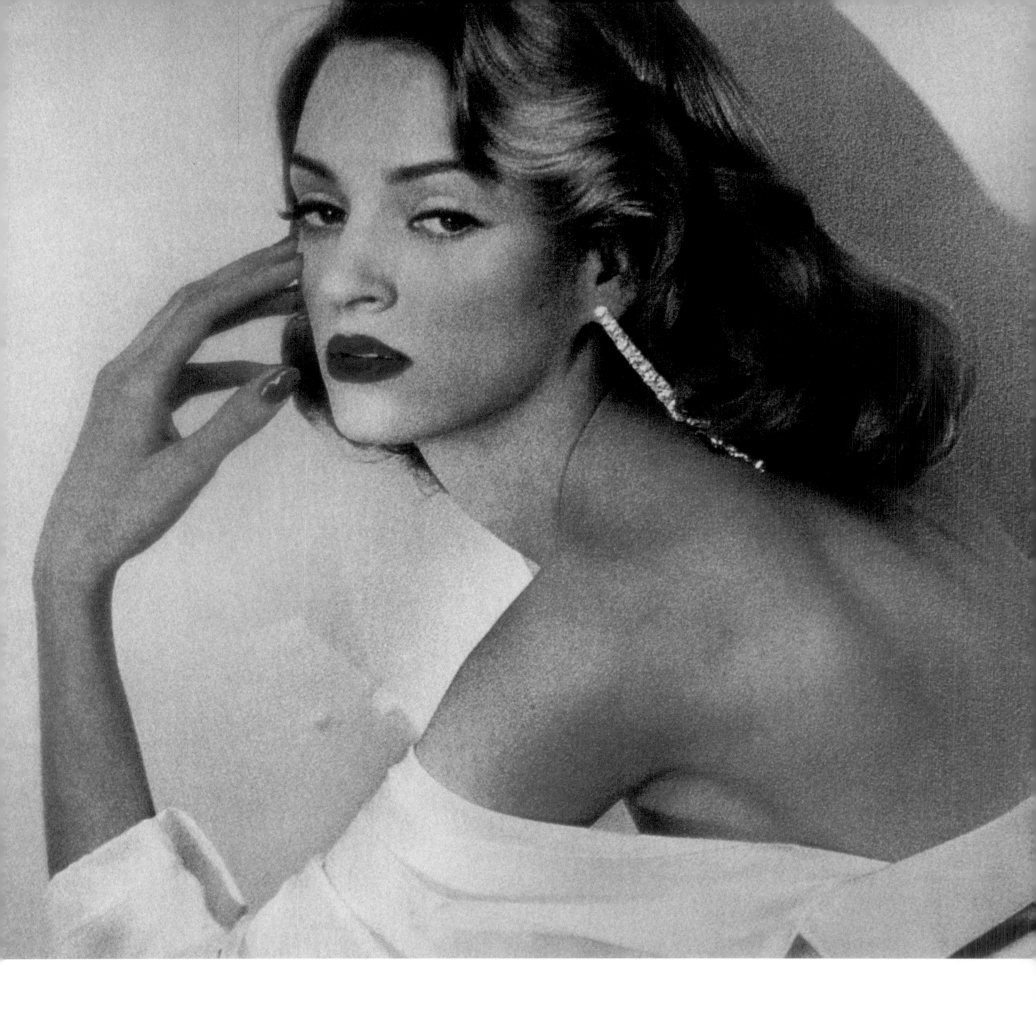

Uma Thurman, photographed by Sheila Metzner for German *Vogue*. Courtesy German *Vogue*

"The ultimate sexy look for the 20th century. This style was coaxed into shape with Thermal Atomized Gel and soft curlers, brushed and then shined with Extreme Spray."

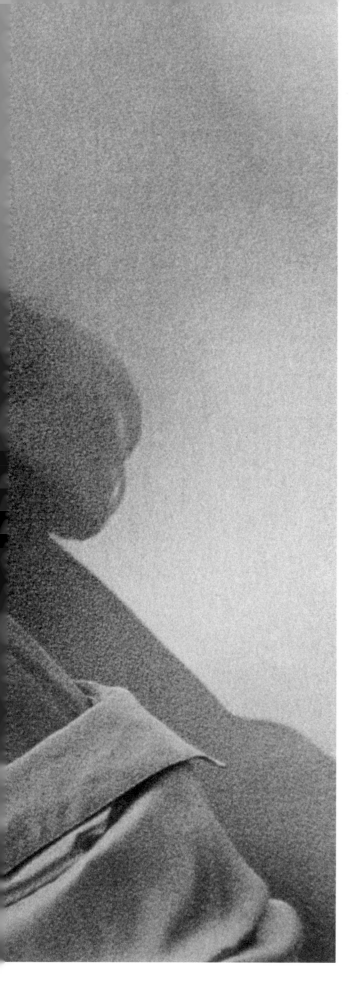

Christy Tur ington, photographed by Patrick Demarchelier for *Harper's Bazaar*. Courtesy *Harper's Bazaar* © Hearst Magazines Division

"Christy's soft romanticism. Gently rippled and rolled with Thermal Atomized Gel."

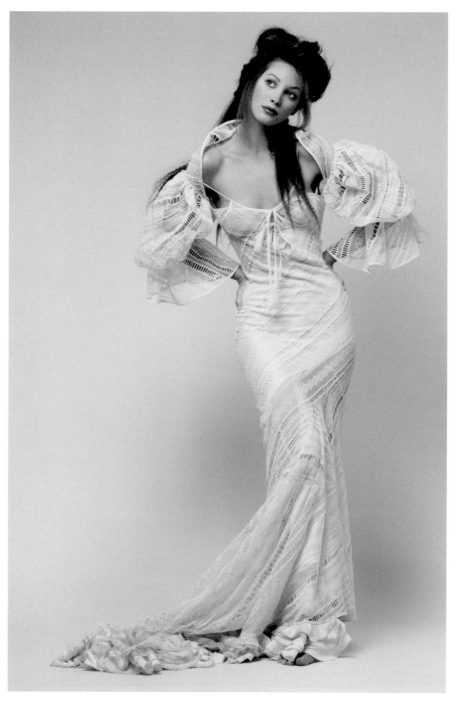

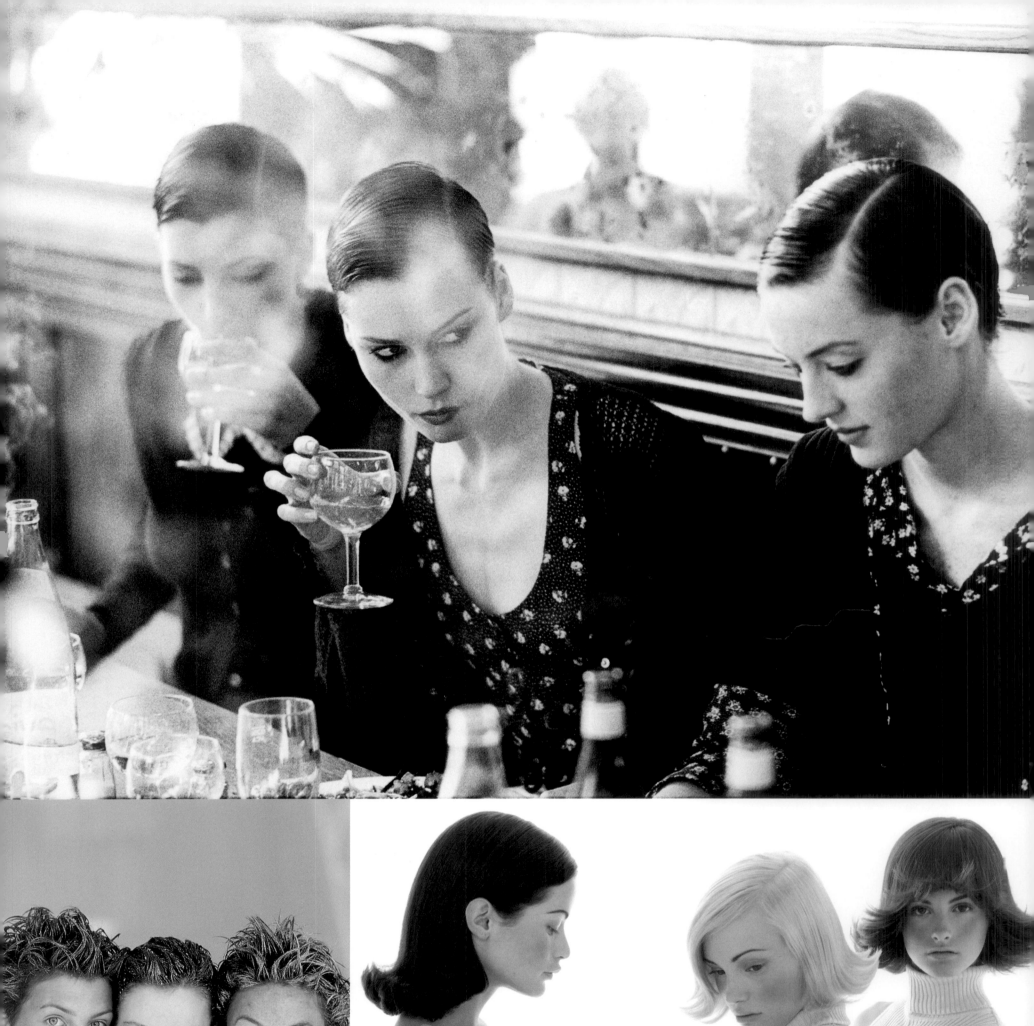
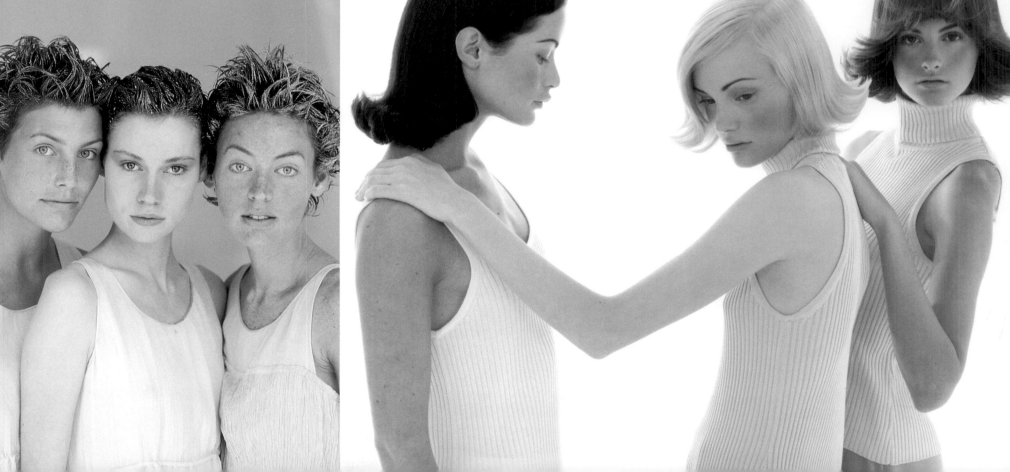

McKnight Rules

As a rule, I believe that one should not be restricted by rules. The only rule in hair that's worth following is to allow yourself total freedom in expressing your individuality. I extend this philosophy to all aspects of life, not just hair. Hair is an extension of ourselves, like the clothes we put on, and reflects who we are. So rather than being a dedicated follower of fashion, be a dedicated follower of your own heart. Having a sense of self, your own intrinsic value and individual sense of style is of paramount importance. The only thing I would say is that if you genuinely care for and love your hair, you will already be making the right choices. That's what having confidence is all about.

"Oh, natural."

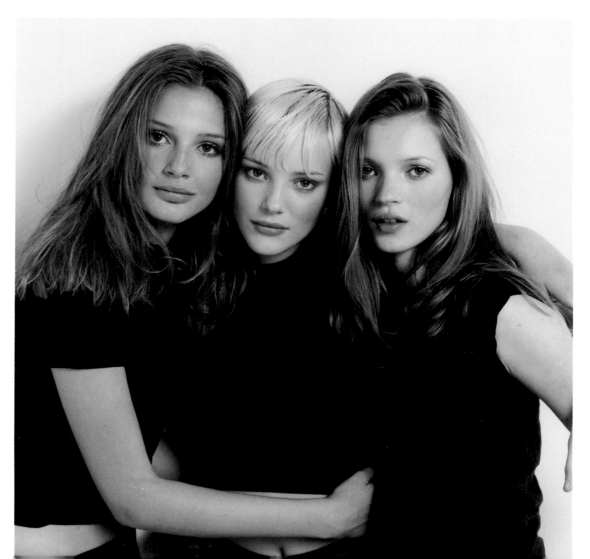

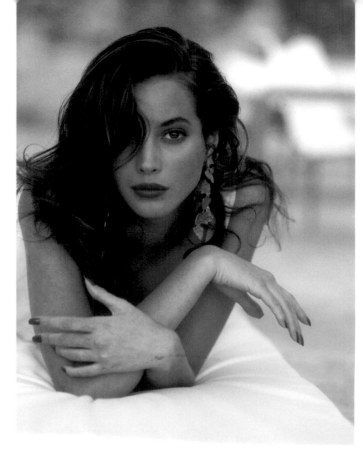

Top: **Christy Turlington**, photographed by Patrick Demarchelier for American *Vogue*. Courtesy American *Vogue* ©The Condé Nast Publications Inc.

"Christy Turlington's relaxed pool-side steamy glam. Steeped in styling base."

Middle: **Kirsty Hume**, photographed by Patrick Demarchelier for TSE Cashmere

"The girl from my home town."

Bottom: **Jaime Richar**, photographed by Patrick Demarchelier for *Harper's Bazaar*. Courtesy *Harper's Bazaar* © Hearst Magazines Division

"Jaime Richar's flip tease. 90s sex kitten, teased, flipped, and sprayed with Extreme Spray."

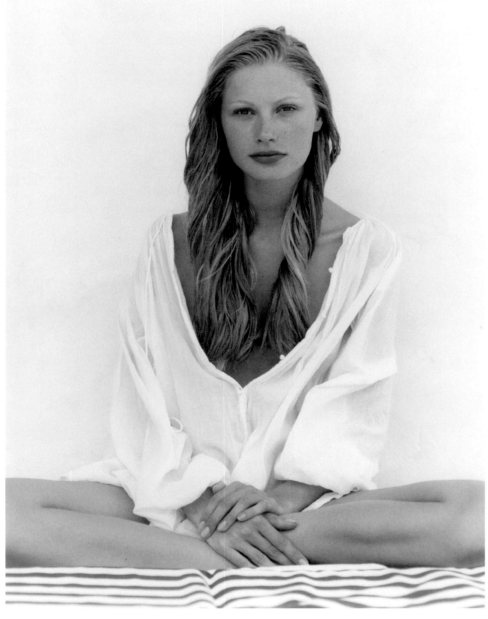

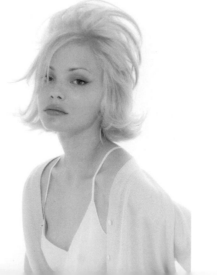

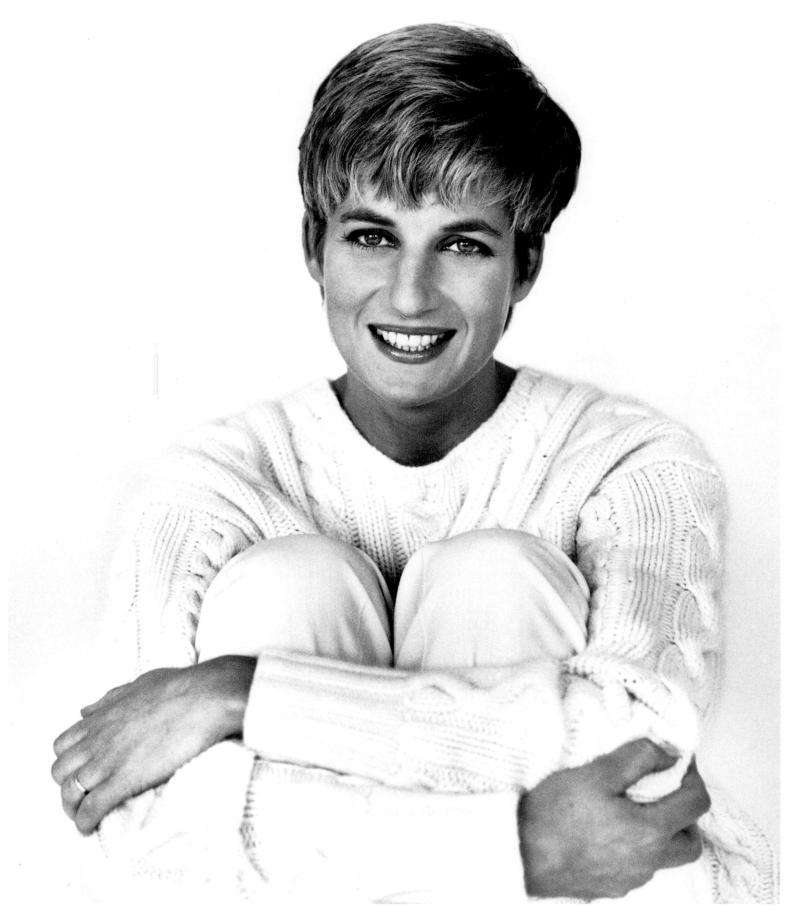

Her Royal Highness, The Princess of Wales, photographed by Patrick Demarchelier

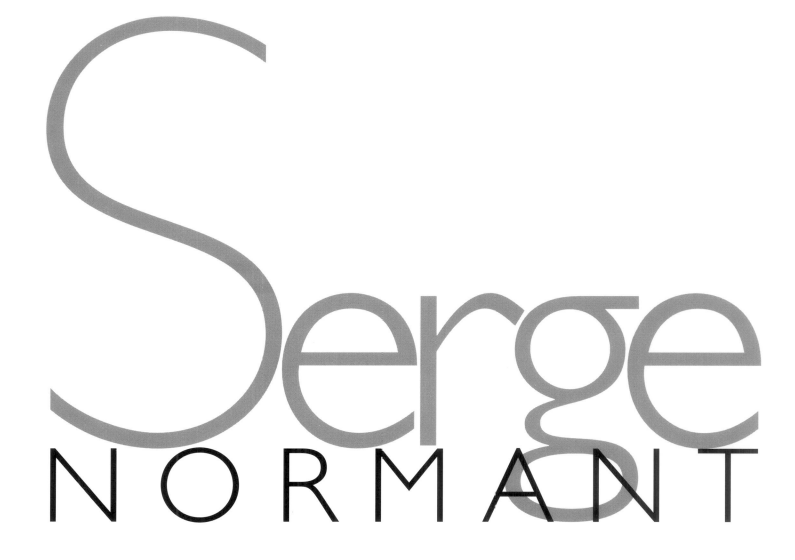

Serge
NORMANT

Sheer Style

Late one brilliant afternoon a single color dominates the Soho studio of photographer Raymond Meier. From two garment racks in one corner of the vast white space hang suits, coats, ballgowns, and dresses in every possible shade of red. Nearby, laid out on a table under the towering windows, is an opulent display of mules, loafers, stilettos, and pumps arranged in a hot spectrum from deep pink and scarlet to tomato and crimson. And seated on a chair before a brightly lit mirror, the flame-tressed model Meghan Douglas is slipping on a pair of long patent-leather boots, shiny as fire engines, which match her glossy Anna Sui suit, textured to simulate alligator skin. While editors from *W* magazine quietly confer and Meier tinkers with his camera equipment in the next room, Serge Normant, the young French hairdresser, fusses purposefully with Meghan's hair. "This is for a Red story," he explains. The group of assembled experts is valiantly trying to wrest some chromatic harmony out of the cacophony of shapes, lengths, and textures offered up by fashion designers for the new season.

Normant has given Meghan a Cleopatra-type Egyptian bob with bangs. It rises to a kind of domed apex at the top of her head, somewhat like the nose cone of a missile. The sides flare out in a pyramidal shape, and the bangs hang thickly over her pale brow, like a heavy shade pulled low over a window. "It's futuristic, graphic, edgy," Normant notes, admiringly. Most of the hair, in fact, is a wig that Normant fashioned and dyed earlier in the day. He then reshaped it on Meghan's head so that it would accentuate her fine, sharp bone structure and compliment the general proportions of her face and body. "Only the bangs are really hers," Normant says. "But the wig is made of real hair." The group now migrates to the room where Meier waits with his camera. Meghan positions herself against the backdrop of white seamless paper and begins striking a series of angular, geometric poses, similar in mood to her red triangle of hair. "Can she swing the hair?" Meier asks Normant. "Yes," the hairdresser replies. And Meghan throws her head from side to side, spreading the red wig into longer, pointier shapes with each toss. The camera clicks, stopping only when Normant steps up to smooth the hair with his palms so the process can begin anew.

Elizabeth Hurley, photographed by Michael Thompson for Estée Lauder Companies

"After applying mousse, I blew Elizabeth's hair dry very smooth. Keeping the front section separate, I teased the rest of the hair up for volume and wrapped it into a French twist. Then I applied silicone to give lots of shine. A classic 1960s look."

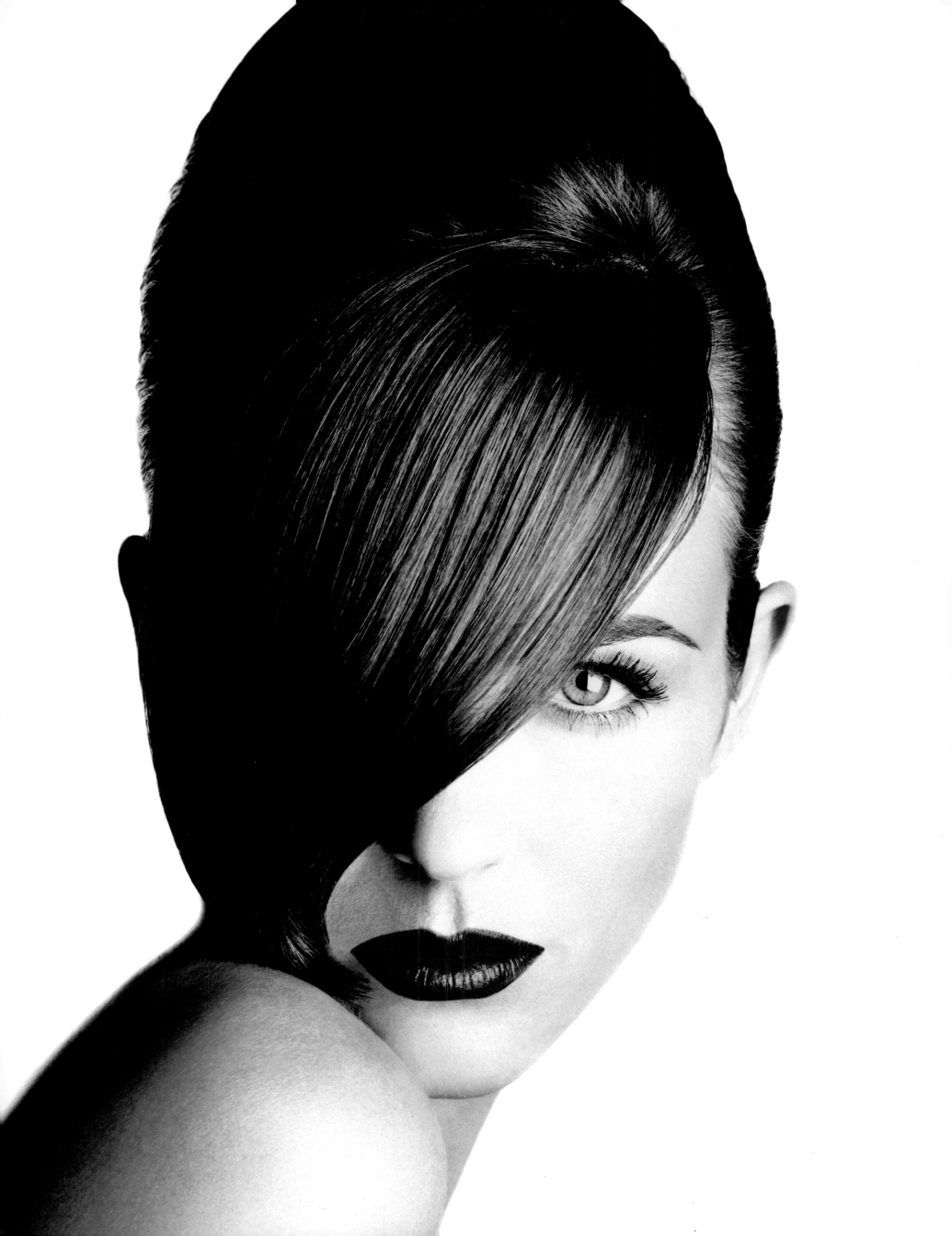

When the shoot ends, Serge Normant loosens a few pins and plucks the wig from Meghan's head, with the kind of gesture usually reserved for lifting a lid off a box. He frees her real hair from its restraining clips and brushes it into a soft, long cascade. Meghan is chattering away about her problems with the contractors who are about to renovate her apartment. "I've given them a 50% deposit, and they still haven't started working. Isn't that dishonest? Oh, Serge," she sighs, "you are honest. You are the most honest hairdresser. You tell me if something doesn't look good. You are a genius." Normant acknowledges her praise by kissing her head.

Average in height and robust in build, Normant is, in spite of his casual attire, a man of very neat appearance. He wears a snow-white tuxedo shirt, opened informally at the throat to reveal some dark, curling chest hairs. He is shod in black motorcycle boots, and he has resourcefully made his faded Levi's into a kind of wearable vanity. In his left back pocket, he has stashed a can of spray; in the right back pocket, he has a brush and another, smaller bottle of fixative. On the edge of his right front pocket, he

has an orderly row of gleaming bobby pins. Clearly, Normant spends very little time sitting down when he works.

For a hairdresser, Normant is unusual in that he is prematurely bald. "I take out my frustration on everybody else," he jokes. The only styling his coif requires is a dot of gel to slick down those few hairs on his pate that would otherwise stand up. "When I first started losing my hair, I had many doubts about my powers of seduction," he recalls in his rapid, lightly accented English. "But all the women in the salon where I then worked, Jacques Dessange in Paris, told me that bald is sexy. For me it is *pas possible* to wear a wig, or comb over pieces that will blow off in the wind, or grow long what I have in the back! No man looks good trying to disguise himself that way. It's never really about the cut or how much hair you have. It's all a question of personality. When you think of Audrey Hepburn, are you thinking just of her hair? I love extreme, powerful looks. For example, one of my favorite looks is a large nose combined with very severe, flat hair pulled off the face. But you need a strong and confident personality to carry that off."

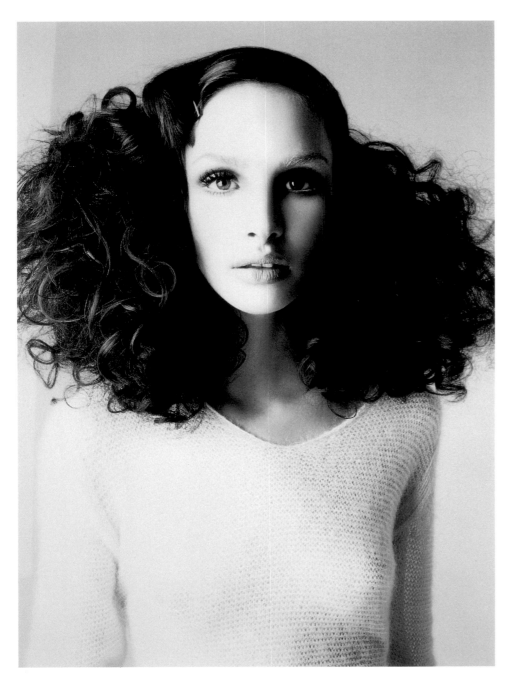

Debbie Dietering, photographed by Michael Thompson for German *Vogue*. Courtesy German *Vogue*

"This very romantic look works because the smooth closeness of the top of the head is balanced by the volume at the sides. Having applied strong styling gel, I curled the hair with a curling iron and put it in pin-curls all over her head. Her hair is naturally dead straight, but with this procedure, the curls stay in all day. I unwrapped and separated the curls from each other with my fingers and a light grease (no brush), then gave her a very low side part, held on both sides with combs."

Julia Roberts, photographed by Firooz Zahedi for French *Elle*. Courtesy French *Elle*

"Using a very small iron, I curled her entire head of hair into ringlets. I parted it in the middle, greased each curl to keep it separated, and then used the same iron in different places on the hair to break the ringlets and create a perfect wave."

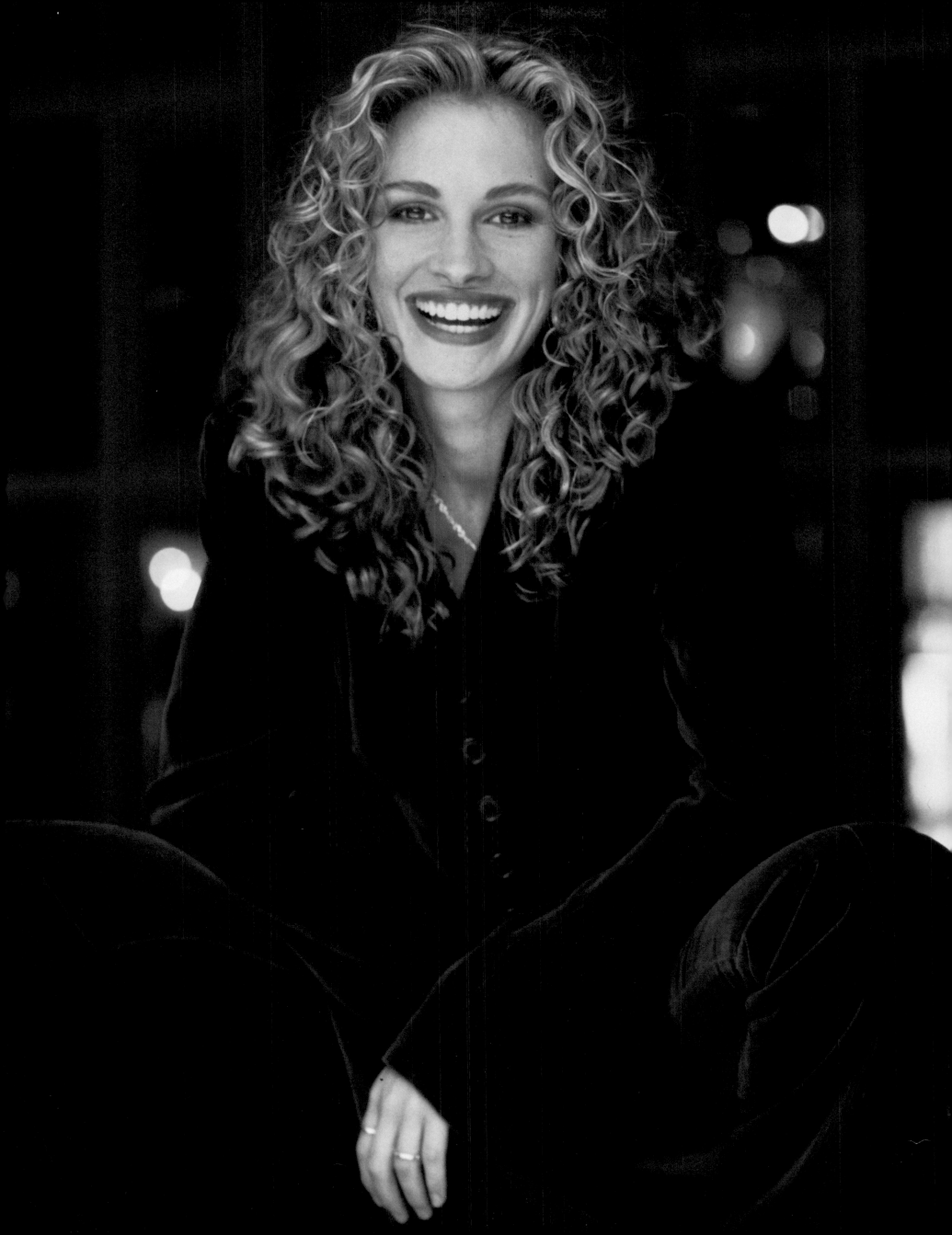

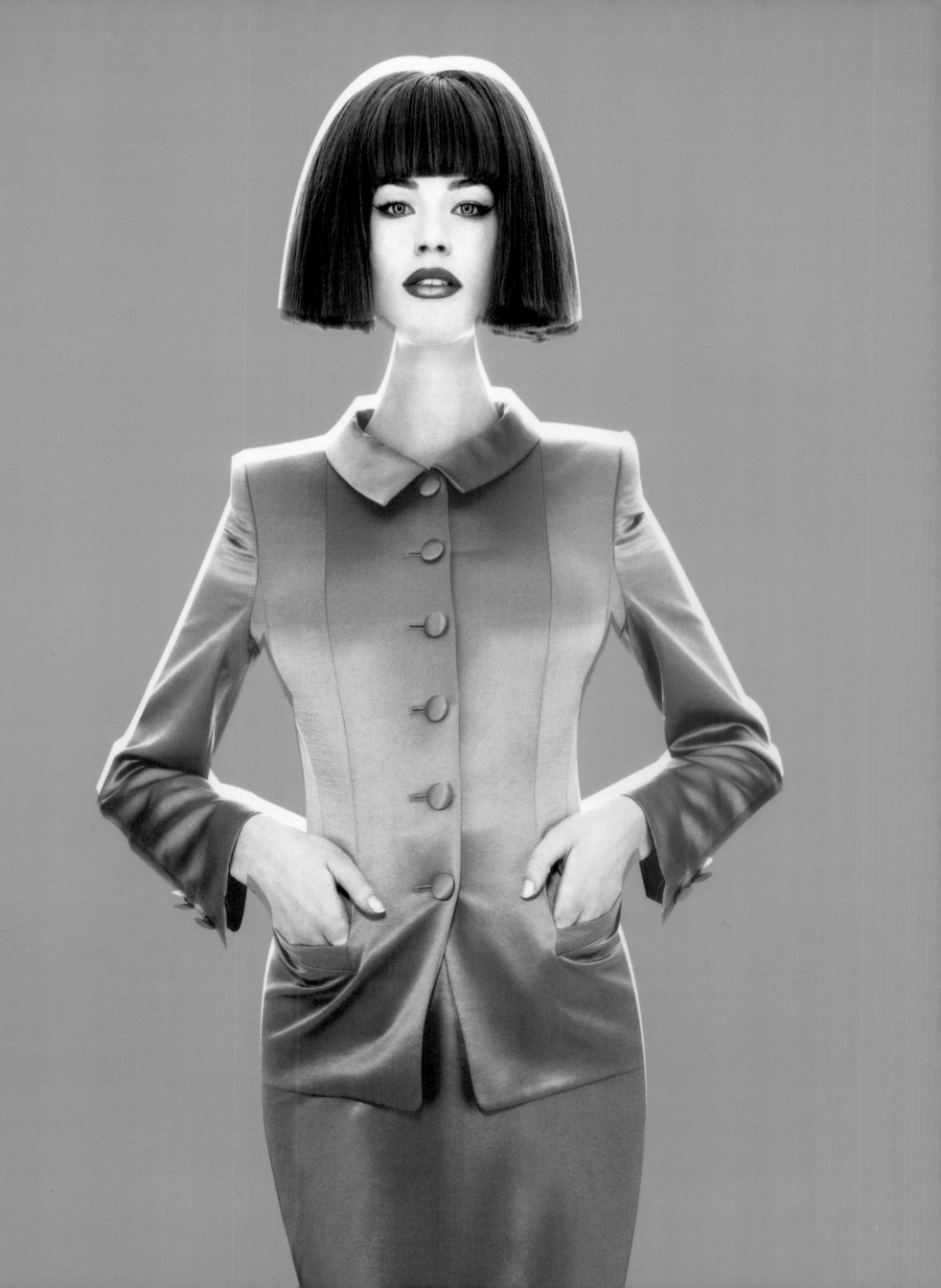

Normant inveighs against the American obsession with "sexy hair and youth," which he feels thwarts expressions of individuality. "It's a real problem here. The fact is, you either look great or you don't — it really has nothing to do with age. Look at Catherine Deneuve or Anouk Aimée in France. I relate to Deneuve the same way now as when she was in *Belle de Jour* almost 30 years ago. Women depersonalize themselves completely when they try desperately to look young! And I hate that saying, 'You look good for your age.' We shouldn't be so scared. Take a chance and be who you are." Normant pauses, his earnest brown eyes lost in thought. "I don't want to blame women for this problem," he continues. "I think maybe it's a question of re-educating men. Can you imagine if I said I wanted to look like Alain Delon? Why should a man think his girlfriend has to look like Cindy Crawford or Claudia Schiffer?"

Instead, Normant exhorts women to find a style that suits their personality. "Look at yourself the way you are. Don't impose another image on yourself, or try to become a copy of some star. All those copies of Farrah Fawcett's hair are terrible — short pieces on top to get crazy volume, long pieces down the side. If you like volume, do it in a way that's reasonable for you. Farrah Fawcett hair looked good only on Farrah Fawcett! I admit it's not easy to find your own style — you really have to learn about yourself. It's a slow process, an evolution." When evaluat-

ing someone's appearance, Normant takes the whole body into account, not just the head. "It's all about getting the proportions right. Short bodies, for example, don't really work with huge hair. There's a right hairstyle for every face and body type."

Normant's reverence for individuality may have resulted from the presence of so many unusual figures in his own early life. He speaks with awe of his maternal great-grandmother, a courageous Vietnamese woman who escaped to Paris with her children and grandchildren in 1959, before Serge was born. "She had white hair pulled into a chignon, and always wore the native Vietnamese dress, similar to the Chinese *Chemsong*. She never learned a word of French because she was already so old when she left her country. I was intimidated but fascinated by her." Another feminine influence was his aunt, a former Miss Saigon. "She was an incredible Eurasian beauty, with blonde Brigitte Bardot hair. I drew a picture of her, which I still keep in my apartment." His father, one-quarter Vietnamese, was an army man who later worked for Air France, and his mother was a fashion-minded woman whose copies of French *Vogue* and *Elle* were eagerly consumed by the young Serge — whose juvenile passions also included Rodin's sculptures, Hollywood movies, and hair. "My fixation on hair did not happen overnight! As a child, I was always chasing my little girl cousins, trying to cut their hair," he says. An avid equestrian, he spent his summers from the ages of 13 to 16 in Ireland, prac-

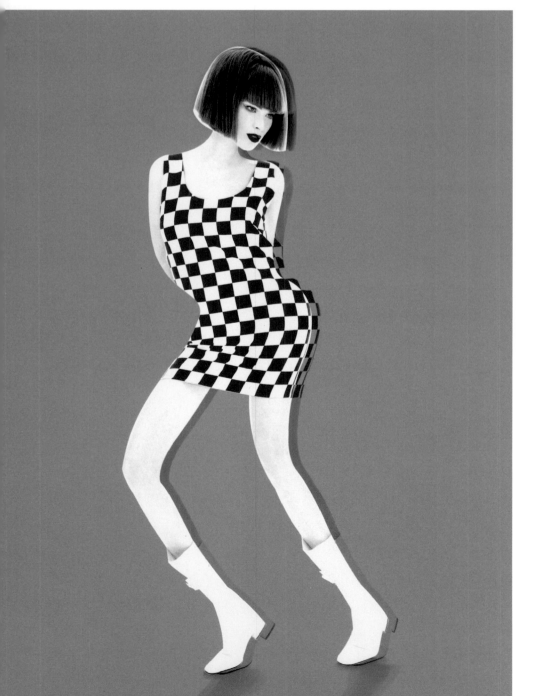

Left and facing page: **Meghan Douglas**, photographed by Raymond Meier for W. Courtesy W

"I wanted a very graphic, Chinese look so I used three wigs sewn together to achieve as much stiff, spiky volume as possible. The bangs are her real hair and the wigs I blow-dried dead-straight before cutting them short and blunt with clippers for this late 1970s look."

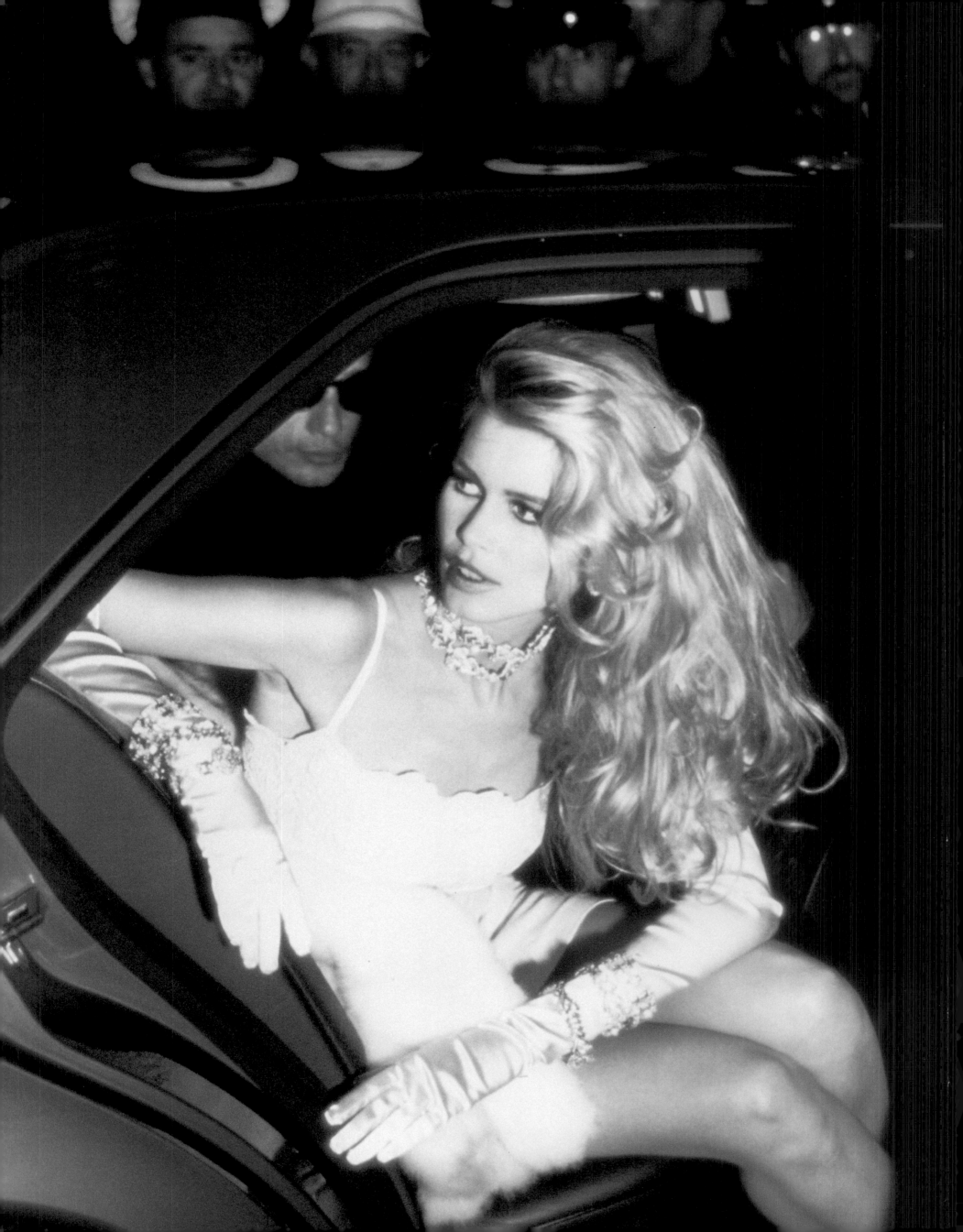

Claudia Schiffer, photographed by Arthur Elgort for Valentino

"La Dolce Vita. I set Claudia's hair on rollers with setting lotion. Once the hair set, I brushed it out into gentle curls and finger-waves to get this effect. Having sprayed with light hairspray and water mist to set the finger-waves, I brushed again gently and added silicone for shine. This is the old-fashioned 50s and 60s way to set hair and it still looks great."

ticing English-style riding and jumping. "As you can imagine, I was braiding horses' tails all the time. Recently, for a show, I braided the models' hair just like a horse's – you do it with two bunches of hair instead of three."

At 17, Normant began an apprenticeship with Jacques Dessange, who – along with Bruno Pittini (Director of the Salon) – was a boyhood idol. "I always loved their work – those edgy Dessange haircuts I saw in magazines of the 70s really inspired me." When Bruno opened a salon in Manhattan, Normant, infatuated since childhood by cinematic visions of American glamour, asked if he could join him there. "In France when I was growing up, America was the dream. To me it meant Audrey Hepburn, Elizabeth Taylor, Marilyn Monroe, Grace Kelly, Rita Hayworth – the sexiest women in the entire world." Though Normant discov-

ered that New York did not entirely resemble an MGM movie set, he was not disappointed. A year before the Bruno Dessange Salon closed, Normant left to freelance as an editorial stylist in the equally seductive dream-factory of fashion. It is still hairstyling's potential for unbounded fantasy that exhilarates him most. "I love the wildest things. Every day is thrilling for me because there are no limits on what I can do. Hair represents everything that excites me – shapes, graphics, touch, texture. I love cutting, I love styling – I love having my fingers in hair. It's exactly like creating sculpture, which influences me more than anything. I collect sculpture at auctions and flea markets. I adore the feeling of clay, and I'd really like to try carving marble with a hammer and chisel. If I ever put this hair thing behind me, I'll definitely become a sculptor."

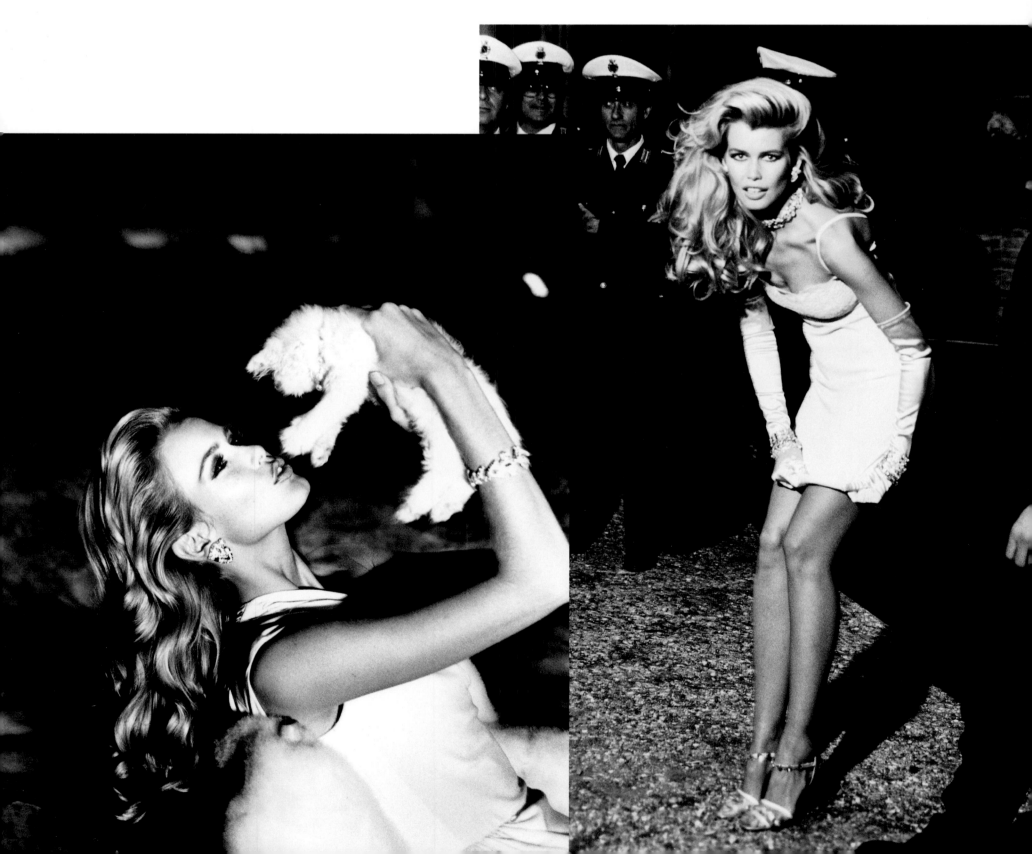

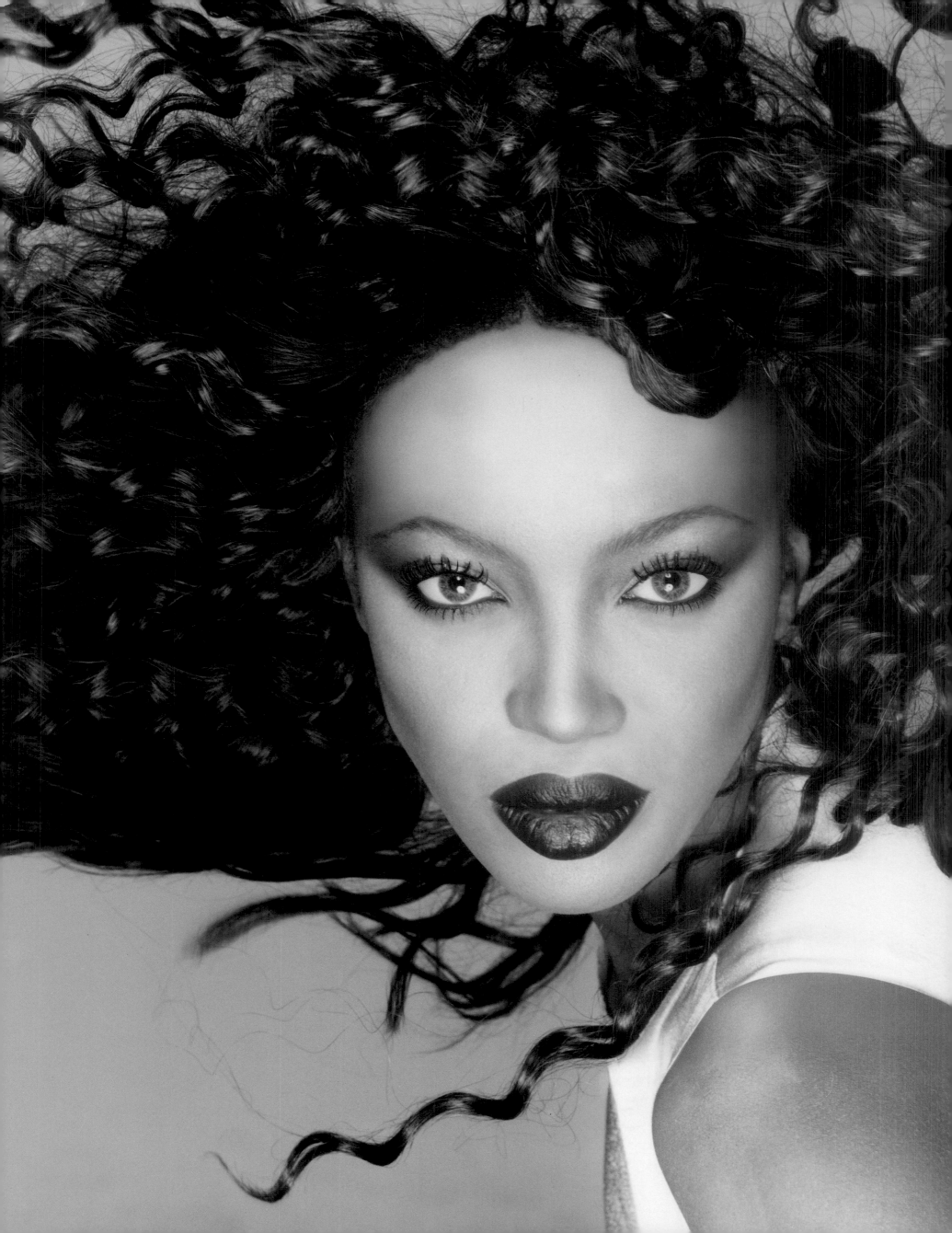

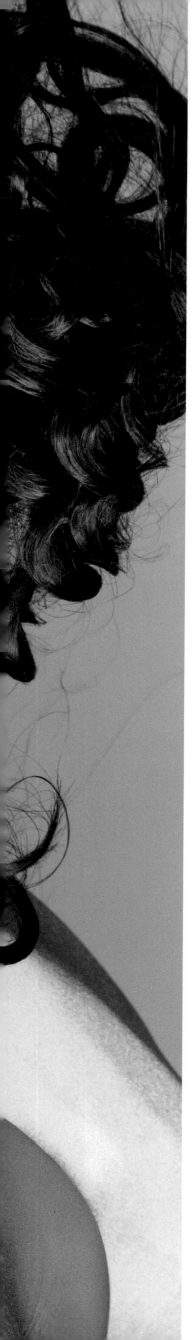

Likes

CUT:
personalized cuts based on facial features and persona

COLOR:
naturally enhanced color based on the individual

STYLE:
eye-catching looks
indifference to age
reliance on personality
wigs
attitude
eccentricity
balance between individual style and trends
sculpted geometric and symmetrical shapes
taking risks

Dislikes

COLOR:
hair streaked with highlights

STYLE:
adopting another's style rather than creating one's own

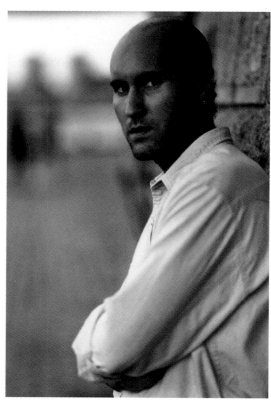

Serge Normant in New York, photographed by Kevin Leong

Hairstory

STYLIST: *Serge Normant*
SALON ADDRESS: *None*
PLACE OF BIRTH: *Paris, France*
FIRST JOB: *Age 15, in a salon in Paris*
TRADEMARKS: *Honesty; Respect for individuality*

Naomi Campbell, photographed by Michael Thompson for *Allure*. Courtesy *Allure*

"I used a crimping iron from the roots to the very tips of her whole head of hair. I left it very loose and used lots of silicone for gloss. A hand-held wind machine created the drama and movement in her hair."

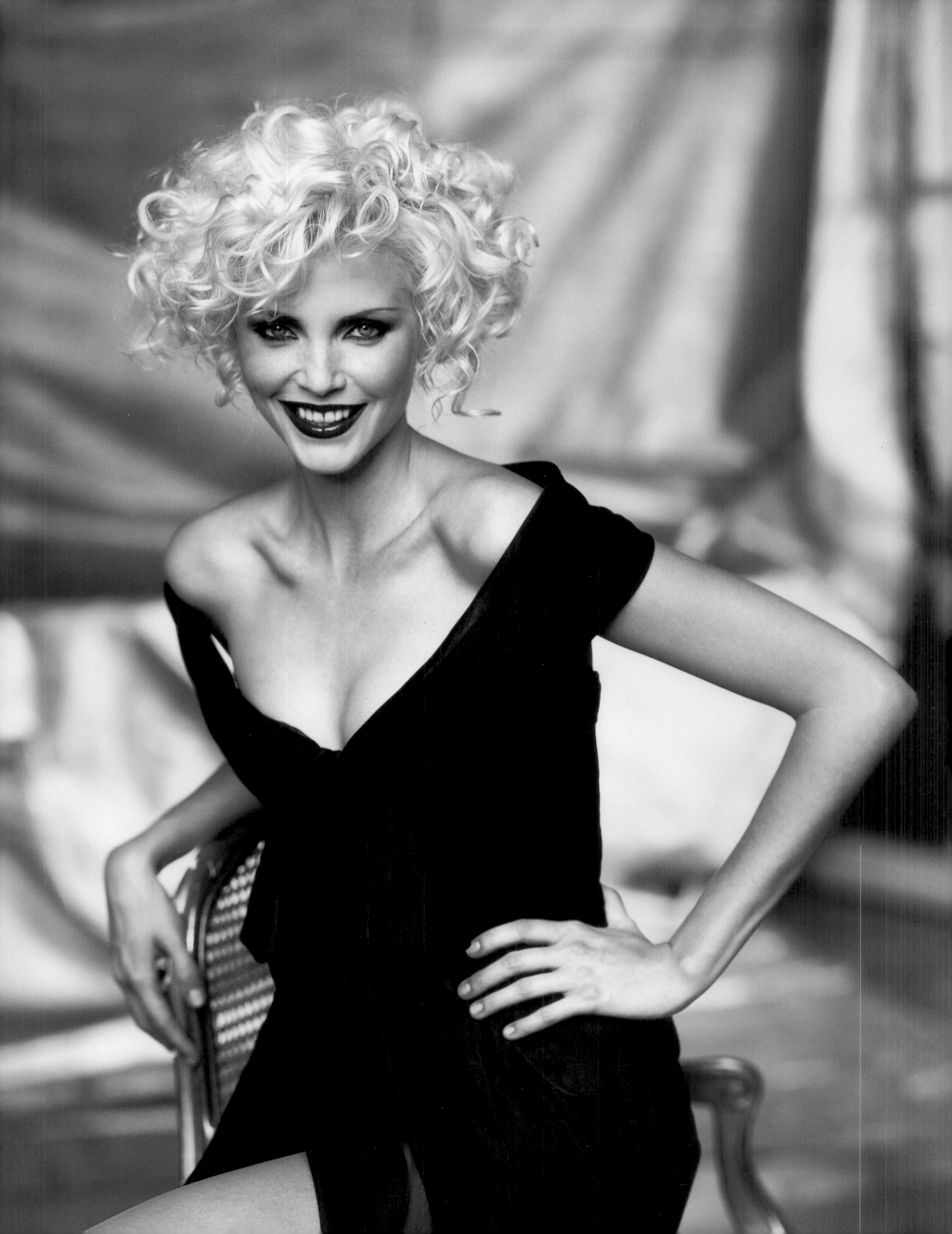

Nadja Auermann, photographed by Arthur Elgort for Valentino

"For this campaign I went for a Marlene Dietrich style. I made an irregular side parting, curled all of Nadja's hair with a curling iron, then pinned hair from the back of her head around her ears in order to give volume to the sides. After this, I used a humidifier at the tips of her hair to loosen the curls a little. Then I added silicone for shine."

Clients

Julia Roberts

Drew Barrymore

Susan Sarandon

Daryl Hannah

Elizabeth Hurley

Helena Christiansen

Kate Moss

Carla Bruni

Christy Turlington

Nadja Auermann

Bridget Hall

Linda Evangelista

Claudia Schiffer

Valentino

L'Oréal

Oscar de la Renta

Anne Klein

Kate Moss, photographed by Walter Chin for Italian *Vogue*. Courtesy Italian *Vogue*

"I wanted an exaggerated romantic look to balance the lightness of the dress. I curled all her hair with a small curling iron and pin-curled it to dry while her makeup was done. Then I unwrapped the curls and separated them all messily. Because the curling had shortened Kate's hair so much, I added an already curled hairpiece for volume and blended it with her hair. I added the fresh flowers as a final touch for softness for a reference to nature."

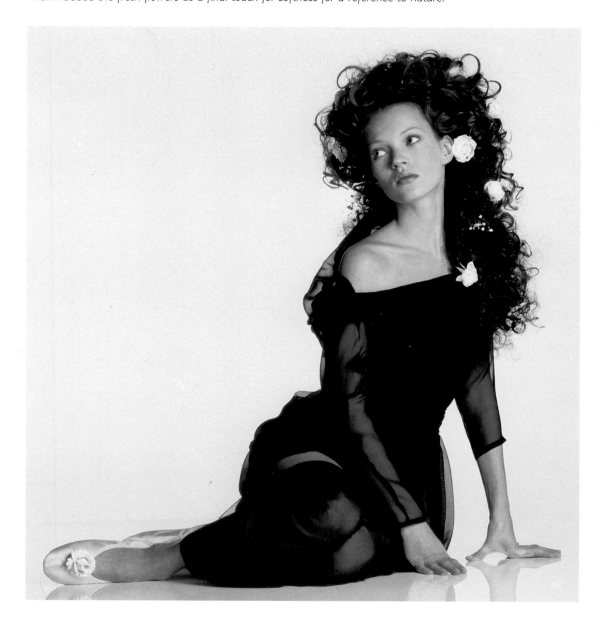

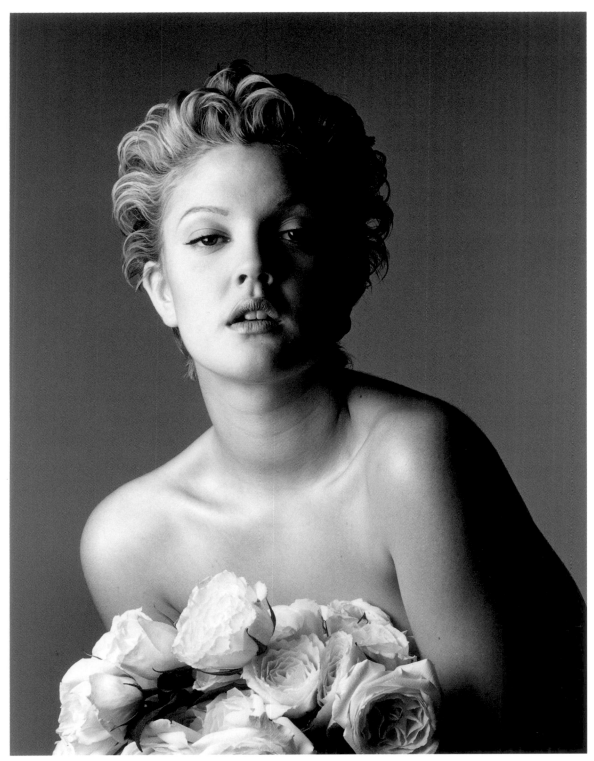

Drew Barrymore, photographed by Bert Stern for *Esquire*. **Courtesy** *Esquire*

"This style is reminiscent of Marilyn Monroe, but shorter. I applied mousse and dried the hair. Then I curled it with a small iron, and did not disturb the curls. I gently greased the hair and set it with hairspray. The curls all overlap each other in a soft and flirtatious style."

Do's & Don'ts

Above all, your hairstyle should reflect your personality.

Take your body shape into consideration when deciding on proportions for your hair. If you are very tall or large, short hair may not work well for you.

When choosing a style, examine the dimensions of your face, especially the length of your neck. The neck is often ignored as a feature and should be shown off more.

The trick to achieving great hair color is to work in harmony with your skin tone. Olive-skinned women should avoid harsh or ashy colors in favor of warm tones. Milky-white skin looks fabulous with red hair. Dark-skinned women should avoid blonde.

Do not use a harsh shampoo; it will strip the hair. Use one with a neutral pH.

Maintain your hair! Have it trimmed every four to six weeks. Use leave-in conditioner regularly.

Massage your head regularly to irrigate the scalp with blood. If your circulation is good and your scalp relaxed, your hair will be strong and shiny.

If frizz is a problem for your hair, use a leave-in conditioner every time you wash, and use grooming products to dampen your hair. A small amount of castor oil works very well for an evening look.

Don't use products that are tested on animals or are overly chemical. There are many great products that are cruelty-free and environmentally safe.

Yasmeen Ghauri, photographed by Walter Chin for German *Vogue*. **Courtesy** German *Vogue*

"This was done for a jewelry story, hence the ornaments. After applying mousse, I finger-dried the hair to bring out the natural waves before adding long, curled extensions. I crimped some of the hair to blur the edges of the style, positioned the front with combs, and loosened some strands around the face for softness. We also used a wind machine to add movement to the hair."

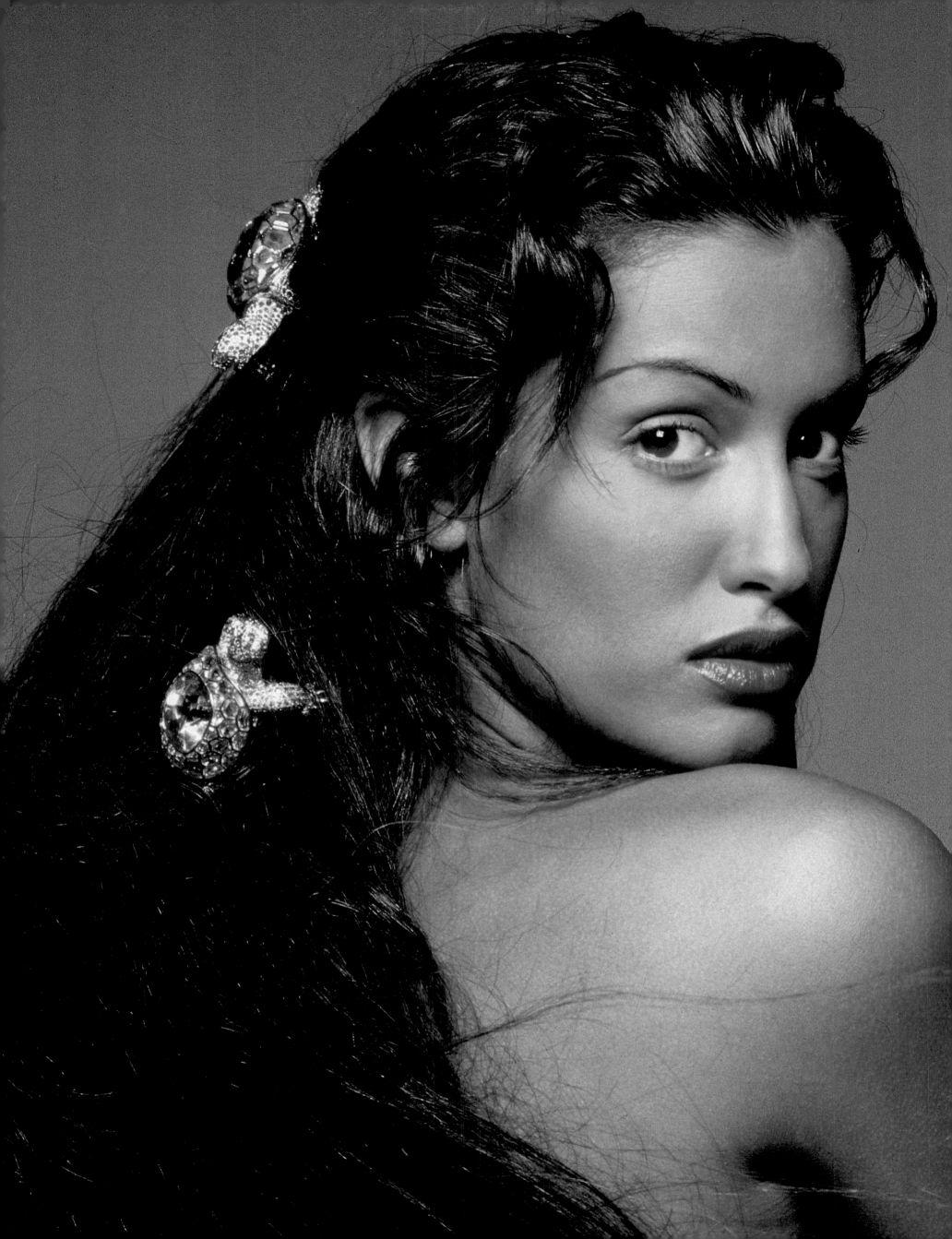

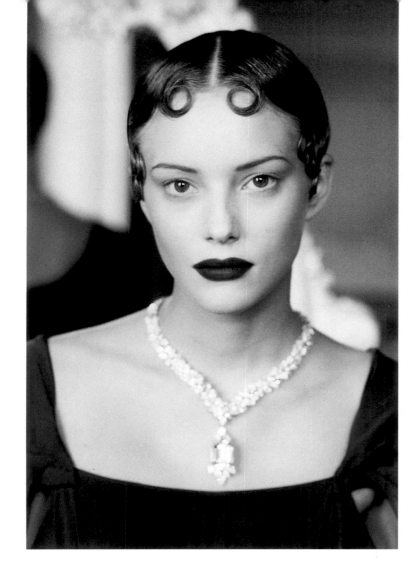

Jaime Richar, photographed by Arthur Elgort for Italian *Vogue*. Courtesy Italian *Vogue*

"This fashion story was on the theme of Josephine and Napoleon Bonaparte. I put her hair in a center parting, gelled and finger-waved it, and left it to dry against her head. It dried perfectly where I had placed it, so I could take out the pins and apply silicone for shine."

Ines, photographed by Walter Chin for Italian *Vogue*. Courtesy Italian *Vogue*

"I brushed down from both sides two triangles of her hair and pulled them into locks. Having put in a center parting, I put the rest of her hair into a ponytail on the crown of her head, half of which I wrapped around the base of the crown; the other half I blow-dried very straight with a slight flip at the end. Her hair is very greased for maximum shine. As a final touch I put in antique hatpins."

Susan Holmes, photographed by Walter Chin for Italian *Vogue*. Courtesy Italian *Vogue*

"This was for an haute couture story. I curled all the hair with an iron, and attached a hairpiece to each side of her head while her own hair was in a ponytail at the crown. I greased all the ringlets to maximize volume for this medieval-type style."

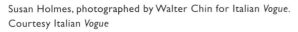

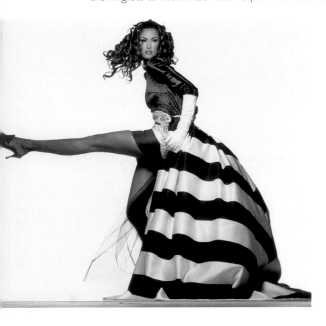

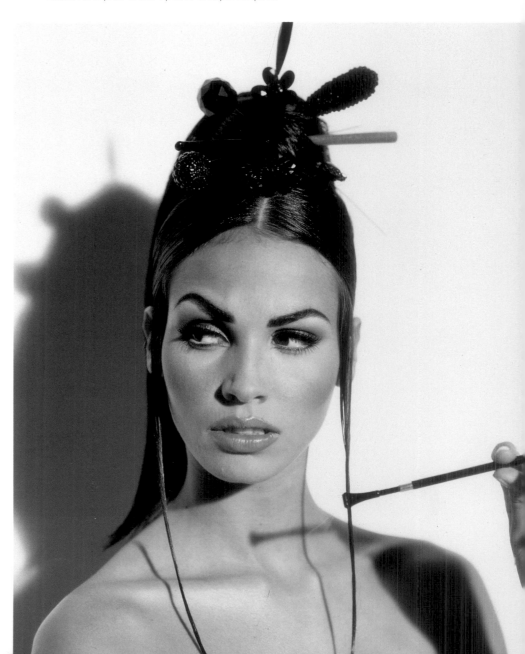

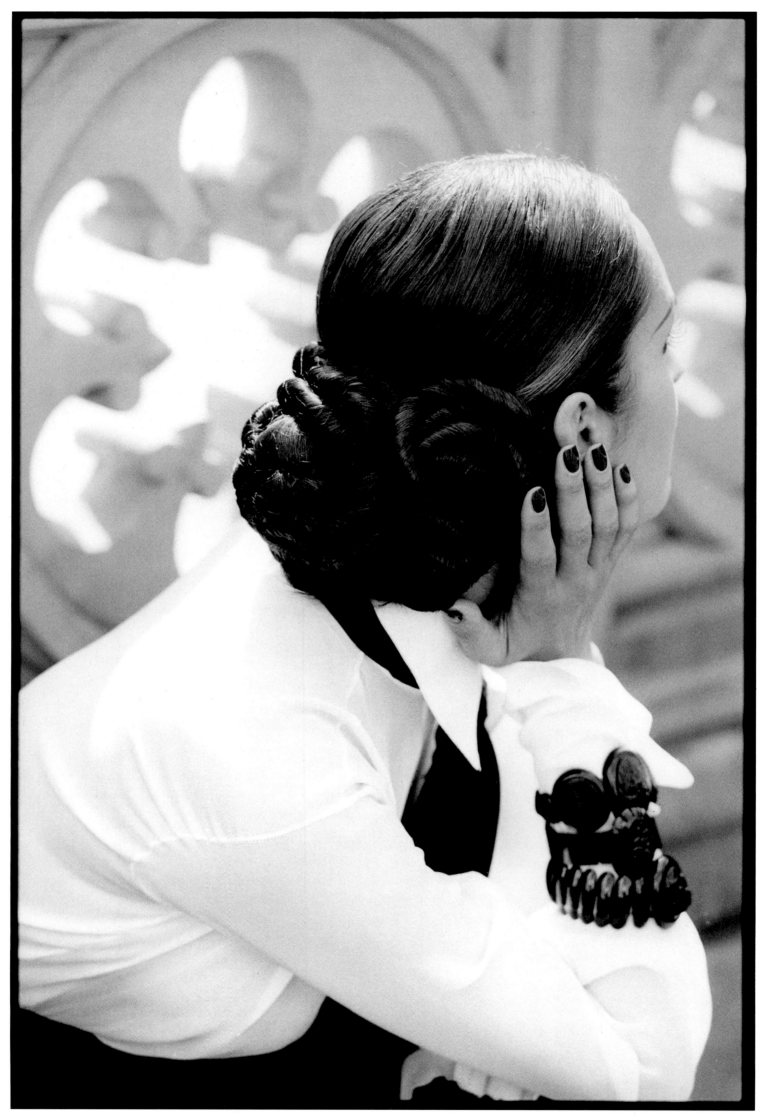

Gayle Elliot, photographed by Patrick Demarchelier for British *Vogue*. Courtesy British *Vogue* ©The Condé Nast Publications Ltd.

"A turn-of-the-century style. I started by adding a hairpiece for thickness, then pulled the hair into a catogan, or very low ponytail. Then, twisting half-inch sections of the hair into spirals and pinning, I created this ornate, yet harmonious, style. The hair has tremendous, spiraling movement, held by invisible bobby pins."

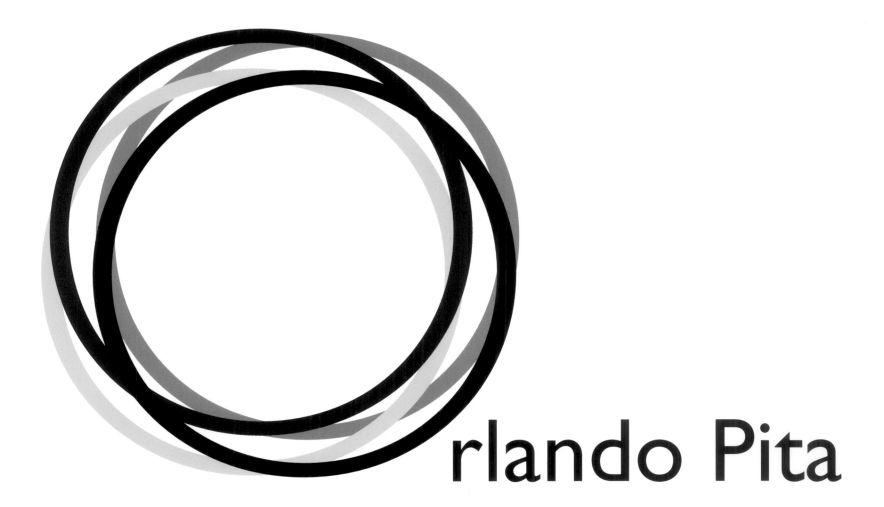

rlando Pita

Something Out of the Ordinary

"The worst thing about people's hairstyles is monotony," says Orlando Pita, the wild *wunderkind* of hairdressers. "The lack of individuality is frightening. Americans are all trying to homogenize, to look the same. This problem goes way beyond hair and fashion, and it's scary."

To the average conformist, Orlando's ideas about hair might seem pretty scary, too. For example, he earnestly believes that "at least once in their life, everyone should shave their head. Why not take a risk and look at yourself in a different way? Hair grows so fast, it's only temporary."

Orlando also vehemently resists shampooing hair – "I haven't for ten years," he admits. Instead, he recommends a clear-water rinse combined with a gentle oil massage. He arrived at this unorthodox approach when his hair grew back curly after he shaved it off the first time. "The curls looked terrible after washing. I left my hair dirty for three weeks and it looked much better, but I still didn't know what to do." Finally, he consulted a South American hairdresser who told him that in Colombia, the Indians believe that hair, like fur, washes itself. According to this theory, regular shampooing accelerates the scalp's oil production. But when sudsing ceases, sebaceous secretions normalize and the oils revert to their natural cleansing function. Orlando convincingly claims his shampoo-free prescription has both cured psoriasis and tamed unruly curls.

Orlando is equally wary of chemically altering color and texture. "You really should work with – not against – what you have. I like gray hair. It doesn't say 'old' to me. If you do use color, make it obvious. I hate little, subtle highlights that are supposed to 'soften up the face.' What does that mean? It's crap! You can soften up your own face – with your attitude, not with dye. It's just a way to force people to spend money."

Phoebe O'Brien, photographed by Michael Thompson

"I enjoy working with braids. I encounter endless possibilities with them."

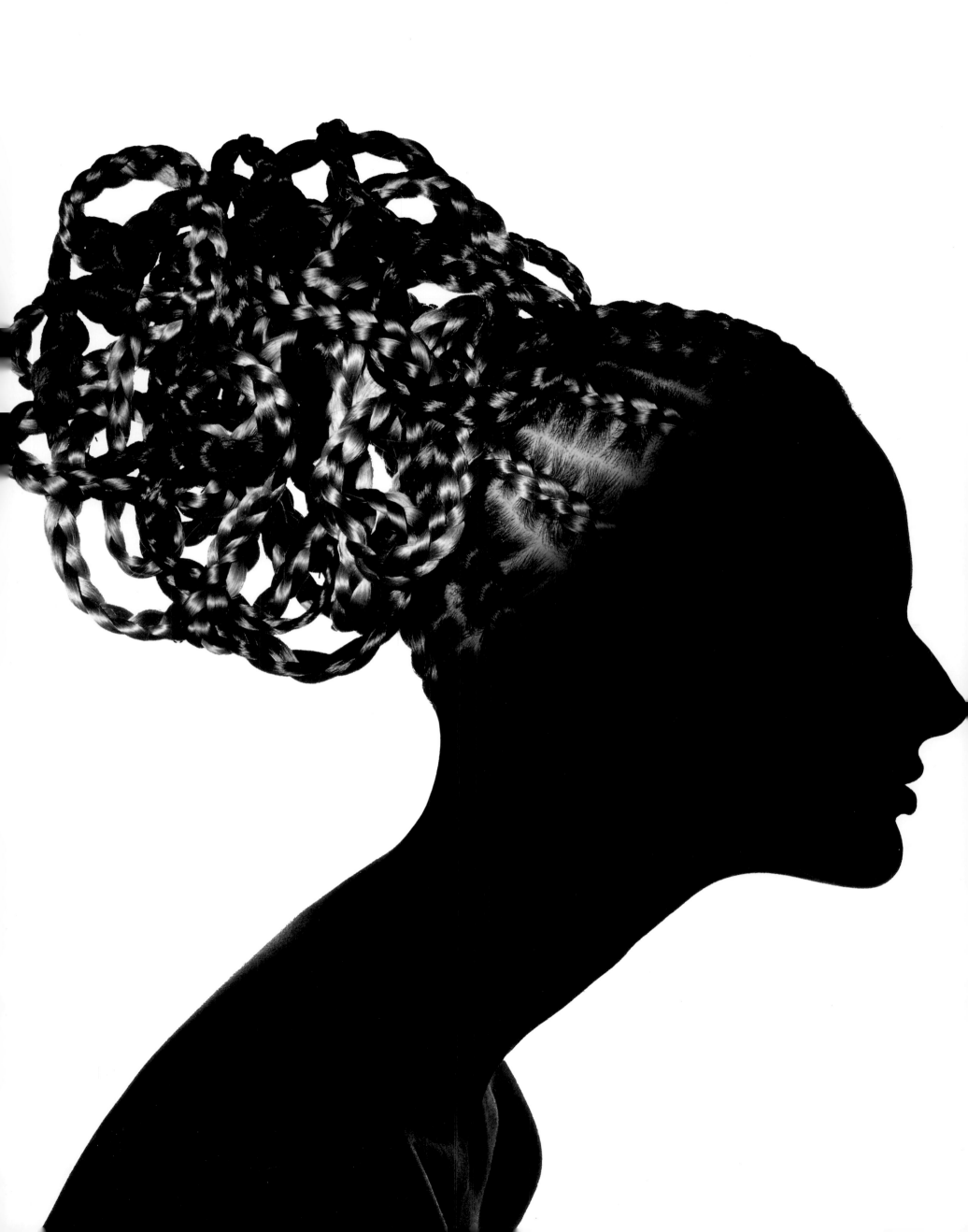

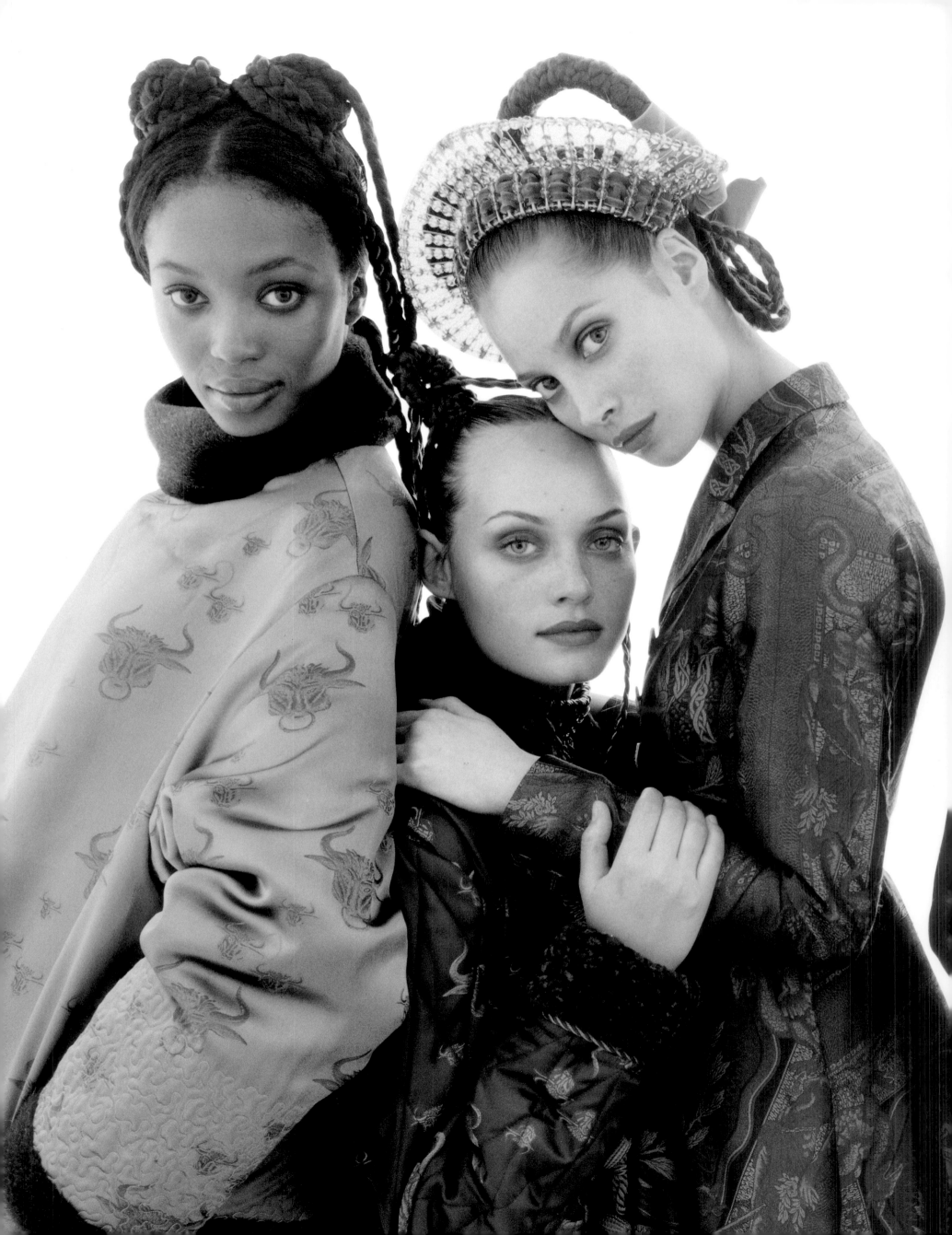

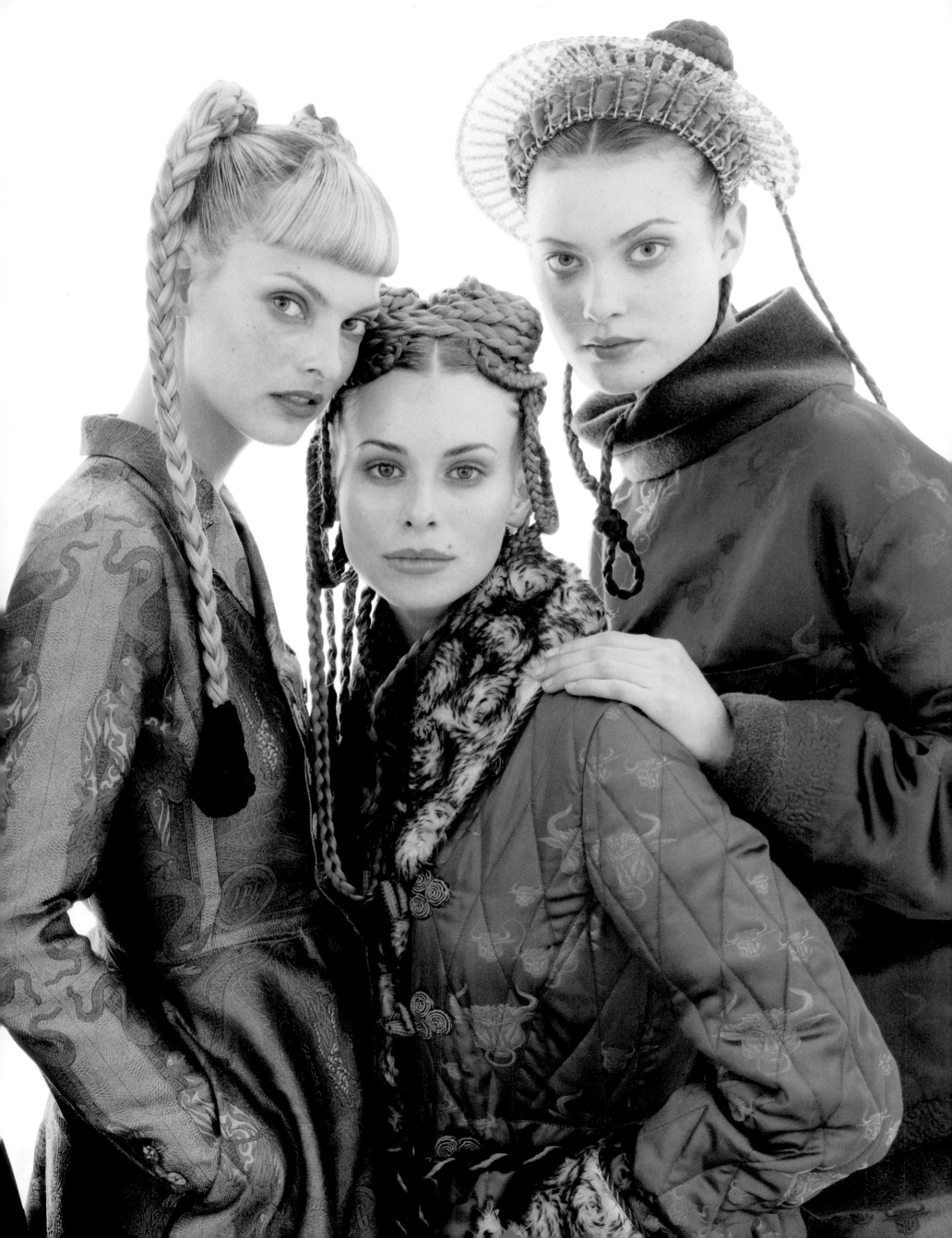

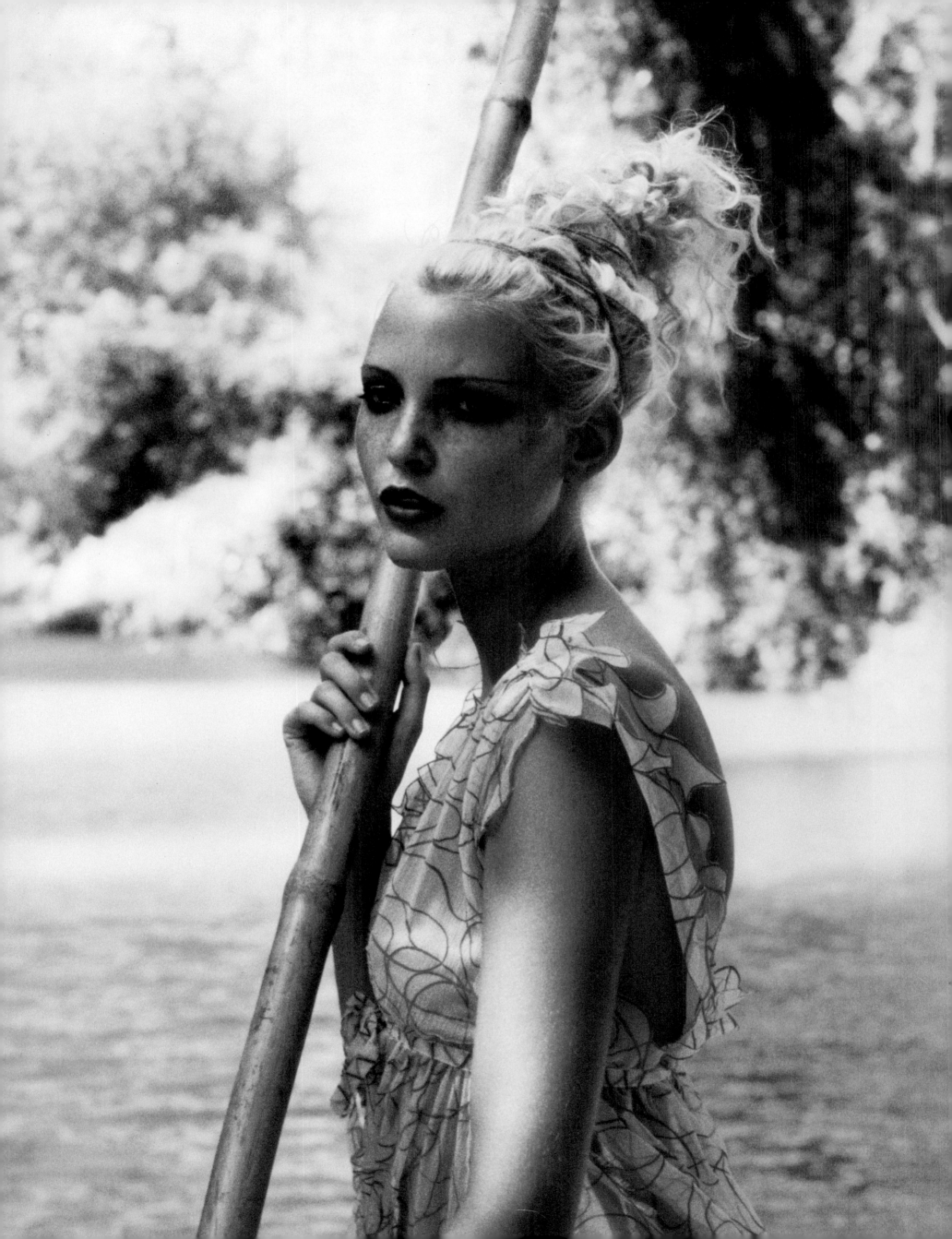

Hairstory

STYLIST: *Orlando Pita*
SALON ADDRESS: *None*
PLACE OF BIRTH: *Havana, Cuba*
FIRST JOB: *Age 12, sweeping a factory floor*
TRADEMARK: *Surrealist, ethnic styles*

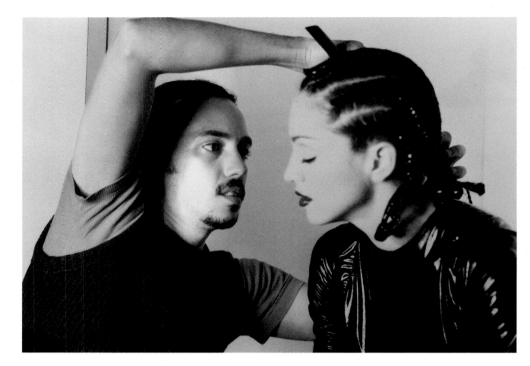

Orlando Pita with Madonna, photographed by Lorraine Day, for her music video *Human Nature*. Courtesy Warner Bros. Records

Previous pages: Naomi Campbell, Amber Valetta, Christy Turlington, Linda Evangelista, Niki Taylor, and Shalom Harlow, photographed by Steven Meisel for American *Vogue*. Courtesy of American *Vogue* ©The Condé Nast Publications Inc.

"I was inspired by the Eskimos, who wear two simple braids, but I elaborated on this style."

Orlando's subversive ideas are an inevitable outgrowth of the startlingly iconoclastic work he produces. "People come to me looking for something strong, something out of the ordinary," he says, understating the case slightly. In his hands, hair is an infinitely malleable material, like clay or fabric, that can be twisted into animalistic textures, such as his "Persian lamb curls," or molded into swelling fruit-like shapes, such as his surrealistic "hair balls," or wrapped around a hardware armature to create coxcomb-like head sculptures. He has even stitched hair into tendril-like spirals and, in his "hair turbans," merged hair with millinery. Fearful of becoming a victim of retromania, he avoids researching hair history and instead takes his inspiration from street looks ("public transportation is the best"), particularly ethnic styles. Hasidic *payos,* Rasta dreadlocks, and African-American braiding have all been reworked by Orlando (often for Jean-Paul Gaultier's runway shows) into novel, head-crowning marvels that bear about as much similarity to a salon hairdo as a Giacometti sculpture does to a department-store mannequin. "I'm in a field where I'm allowed to do what I like," says Orlando, who stopped seeing clients two years ago in order to concentrate solely on session work. "It doesn't really relate to real life. I always have an end picture in mind – whatever it takes to get there, I'm willing to try it. It's all about fantasy, dreams, and inspiration."

Orlando has had enough "real life" experience to understand the necessity of dreams. To improve their economic circumstances, his family left Cuba in 1967 for West New York, New Jersey, where his father found work at a knitting mill. His mother sewed clothing for herself and her three sons out of fabric brought home from the factory. "I learned to sew by watching her," he says. Every Saturday she went to the beauty salon on the corner to have her hair arranged in "a huge beehive hairdo," Orlando recalls. "It would last all week." His mother fascinated him with stories about friends who stashed valuables inside their bouffant 'dos when fleeing Cuba during the revolution. Orlando's grandmother, who arrived in 1972, "gave me insight into a world that my parents would never have exposed us to. She brought my brothers and me to the museums and parks of Manhattan" – whose skyline loomed, like a beckoning Emerald City, over West New York. "All of us ended up in the arts," Orlando says. "We all rebelled."

One of Orlando's earliest rebellious acts was to take an after-school job. "At age 12, I was cleaning a sewing factory for minimum wage – $2.00 an hour. It was against my parents' wishes, but it felt like freedom to me. I spent the money on records and clothes." More janitorial work followed, at a grammar school and a pharmacy. By age 15, he was escaping to Studio 54, staying up all night, and sleeping only when he returned from school at 3 p.m. Miraculously, he was still able to perform well academically. "I had a quick mind, especially for math. And I wasn't too challenged," he says. Orlando eventually quit school, moved out of the family

Nadja Auermann, photographed by Ellen von Unwerth for American *Vogue*. Courtesy American *Vogue* ©The Condé Nast Publications Inc.

"I wanted to make Nadja look like a goddess."

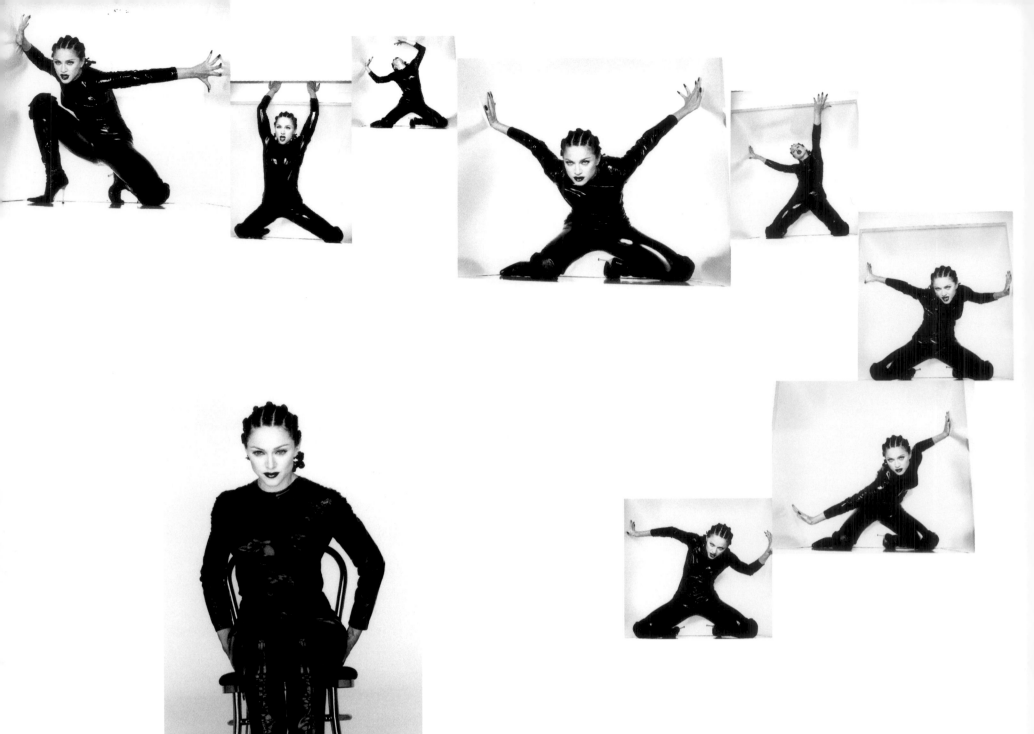

home, and began commuting to various low-paying jobs in Manhattan. For one Wall Street company he redeemed stocks and bonds, and for another, an insurance firm, he invested funds. Weary of drifting from one dull job to another, he packed up and moved to Florida, where he knew no one. "It was tough, but I wanted to change my life. The year and a half I spent there taught me some very good lessons." He worked in a hospital admissions office, where he assigned patients to wards according to their diseases. Throughout these restless years, from the age of 14, Orlando had also been cutting hair on the side. "Once I gained enough confidence, I even started charging – I was always a little businessman. But I never wanted to work in a salon. I hated the awful, catty atmosphere I had seen there, so I never considered making hairdressing my profession. It hadn't occurred to me that you could be a hairdresser without a salon."

The Florida adventure having run its course, he called his brother José, a photographer's assistant living in Brooklyn, and asked if he could move in with him. One day, the photographer's hairdresser cancelled half an hour before a shoot, and José persuaded his brother to fill in. Orlando reluctantly showed up at the studio, clutching a brown paper bag full of drugstore products. "Everybody thought it was very funny," he recalls. When the photographer's agent saw the results of this impromptu session, she found more than humor in the situation. In fact, she offered to represent Orlando for a six-month trial period. "She thought I had talent," he says.

In November 1984, he arrived in Paris, invited by another agent who had been similarly impressed by the fledgling studio stylist's work. One week later, Orlando was booked by Peter Lindbergh, and before long he was also doing runway shows for

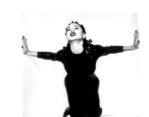

Madonna, photographed by Lorraine Day for her music video *Human Nature*. Courtesy Warner Bros. Records

"I developed this style as a way of covering her blonde hair and making it look dark. I sewed patent leather into the braids, which took nearly four hours, but she was very patient."

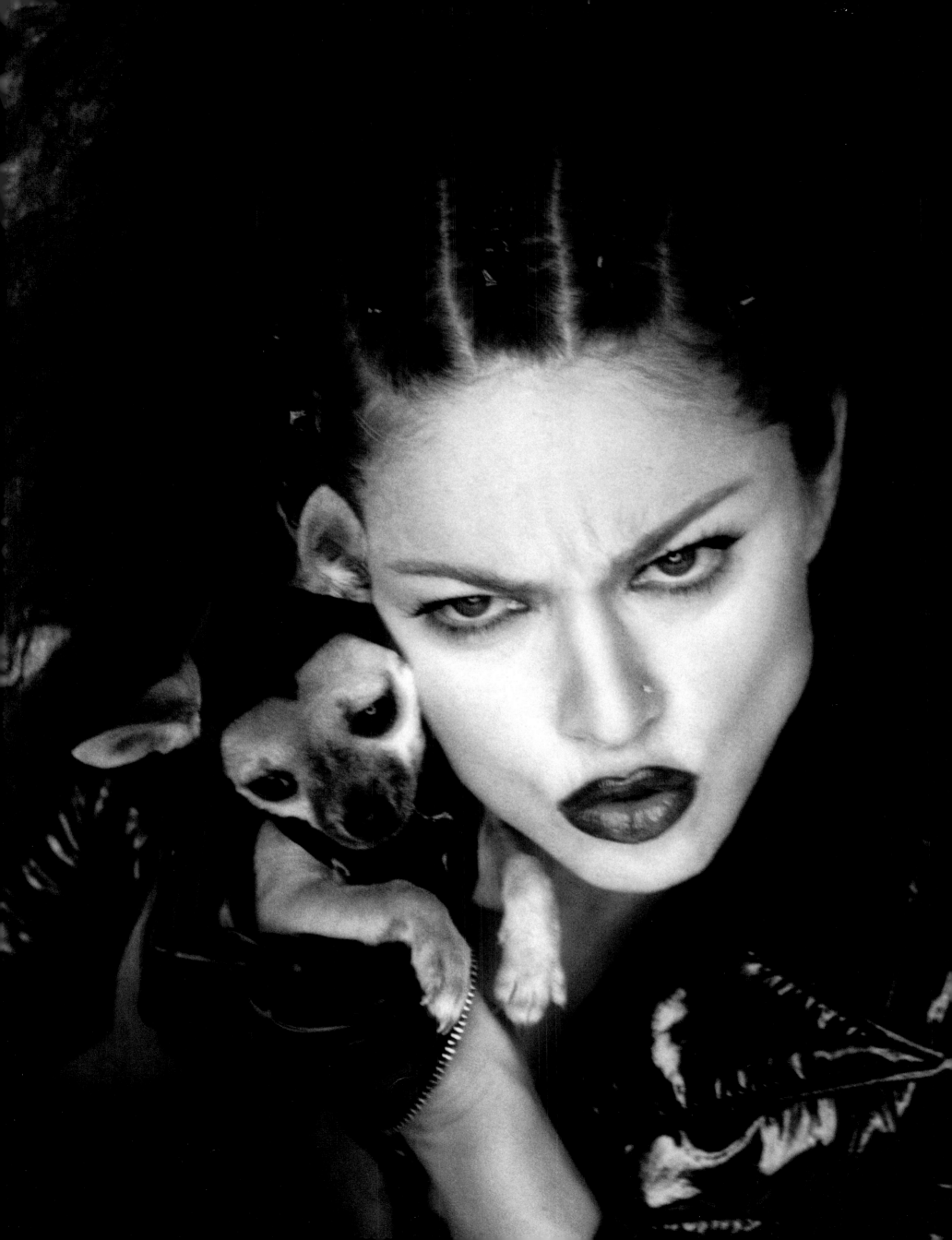

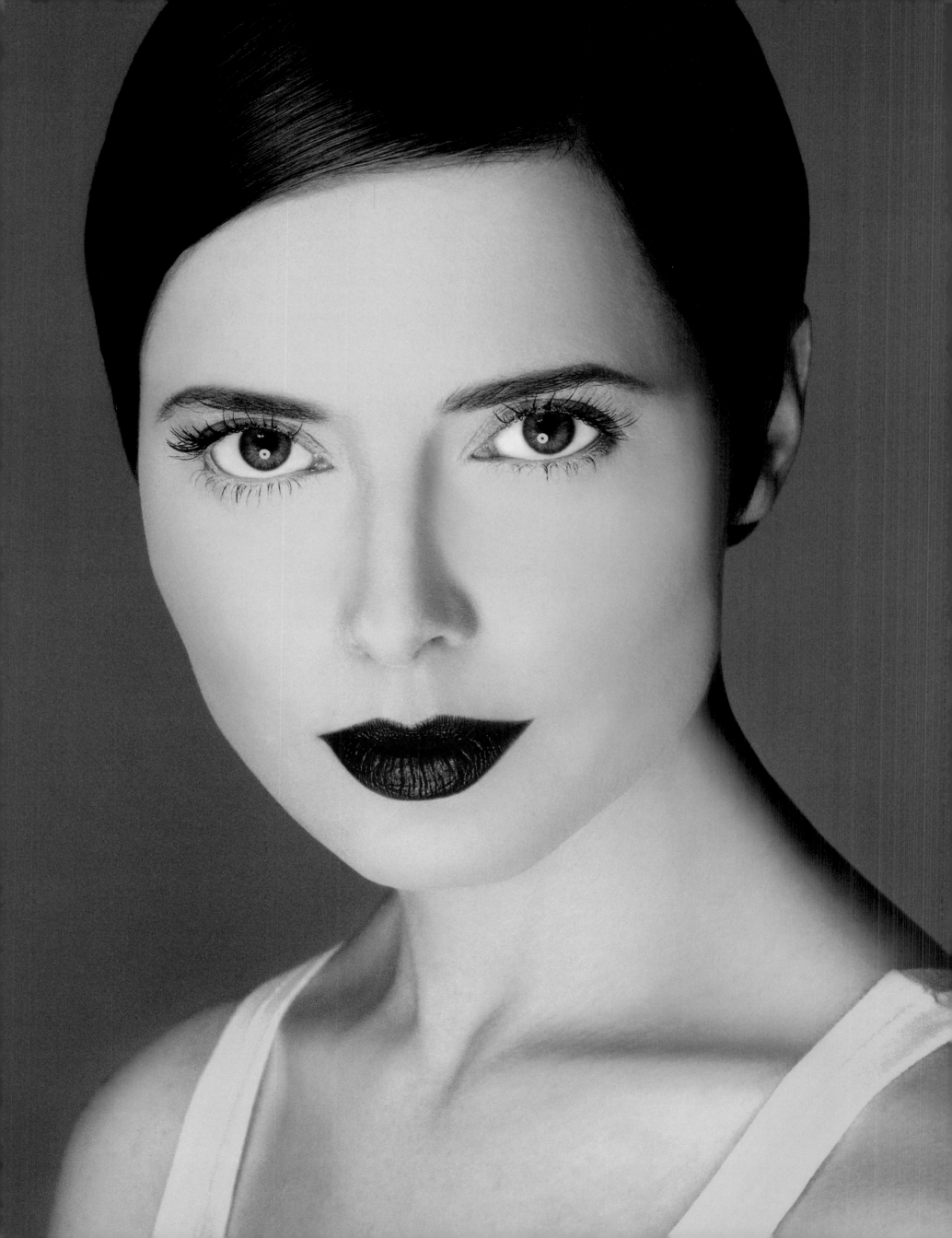

Martine Sitbon and Yohji Yamamoto. Three years passed before he felt ready to return to New York. "My first success was in Paris, because the only designers who understood constructed, extravagant hair were there. In America at that time, everyone wanted loose, exercisy, aerobics hair."

These days, it seems, everybody wants Orlando's brand of inventive, oddball style. He travels so incessantly for magazines, advertisers, and designers that he estimates he is home only three or four months a year. And by now he has the career record of someone twice his age. He commanded comb and scissors at Naomi Campbell's first shoot (for British *Elle*), worked on

Nadja before she was a blonde, and fussed with Shalom's tresses before she turned brunette. Recently, Chanel, one of the industry's most coveted accounts, has taken him on for both ads and shows. And Madonna now depends on him for personal haircuts and styling on her videos. At this rate, he can easily afford to turn away lucrative bookings if the work doesn't interest him. "I'm not so sure I can keep this up forever," he reflects. "It's very hard on the body. I don't know how someone like Karl Lagerfeld has stayed so enthusiastic about fashion for so long. My dream is to establish a health spa somewhere near a beach. And maybe just keep my mother, grandmother and father as clients."

Isabella Rossellini, photographed by Michael Thompson for *Allure*. Courtesy *Allure*

"Both of these photographs are from a story where six of Isabella's favorite makeup artists did her makeup. I did her hair for each look."

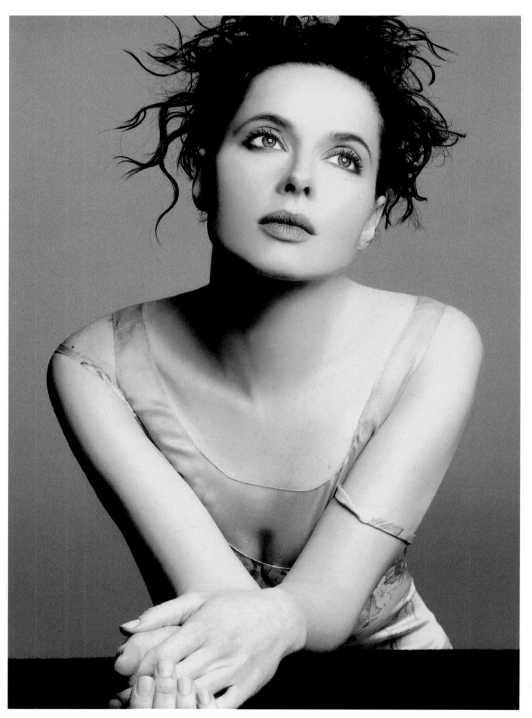

"Here Isabella has a more ethereal and angelic look."

"Makeup artist Kevyn Aucoin created a very clean and pure look. I think we achieved the simple lines he wanted."

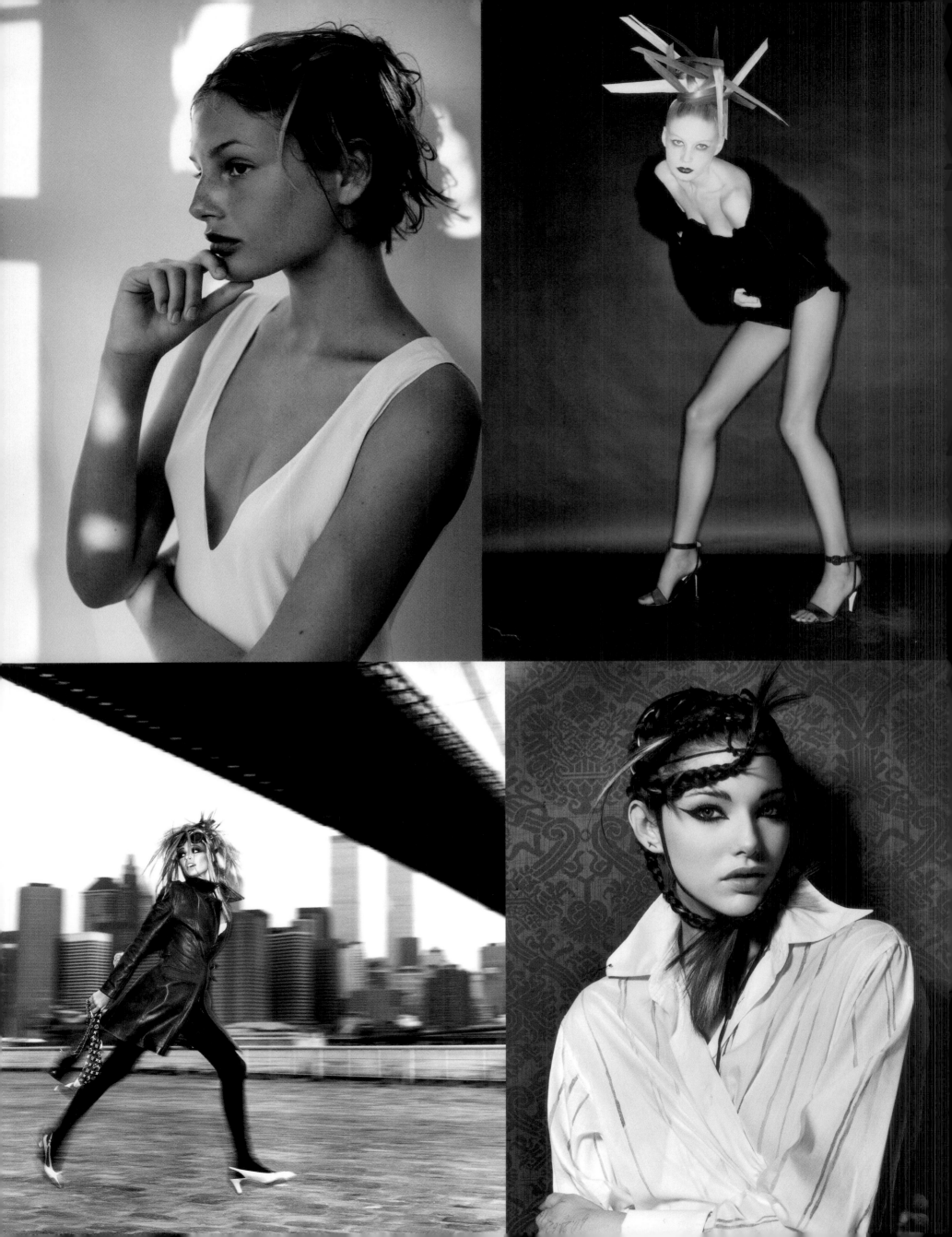

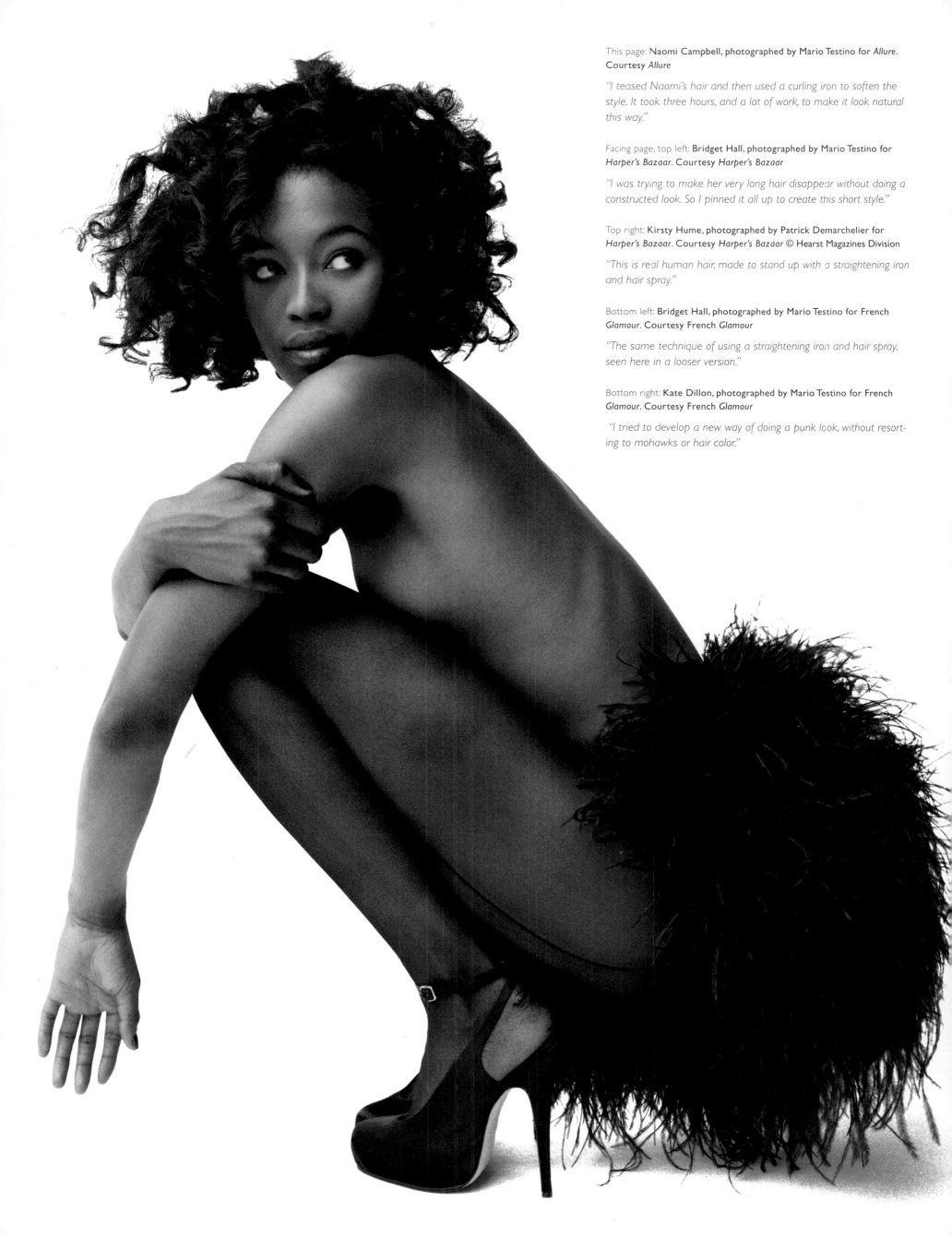

This page: Naomi Campbell, photographed by Mario Testino for *Allure*. Courtesy *Allure*

"I teased Naomi's hair and then used a curling iron to soften the style. It took three hours, and a lot of work, to make it look natural this way."

Facing page, top left: Bridget Hall, photographed by Mario Testino for *Harper's Bazaar*. Courtesy *Harper's Bazaar*

"I was trying to make her very long hair disappear without doing a constructed look. So I pinned it all up to create this short style."

Top right: Kirsty Hume, photographed by Patrick Demarchelier for *Harper's Bazaar*. Courtesy *Harper's Bazaar* © Hearst Magazines Division

"This is real human hair, made to stand up with a straightening iron and hair spray."

Bottom left: Bridget Hall, photographed by Mario Testino for French *Glamour*. Courtesy French *Glamour*

"The same technique of using a straightening iron and hair spray, seen here in a looser version."

Bottom right: Kate Dillon, photographed by Mario Testino for French *Glamour*. Courtesy French *Glamour*

"I tried to develop a new way of doing a punk look, without resorting to mohawks or hair color."

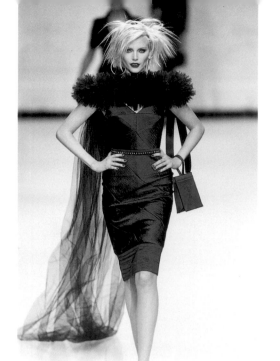

Nadja Auermann, photographed by Patrice Stable for *Salon News*

"I wanted to make the hair look like feathers."

Likes

CUT:
shaved heads

COLOR:
bold, obviously dyed hair
naturally gray hair

STYLE:
African-American street styles
traditional ethnic styles
exotically sculpted hair
anything out of the ordinary

TREATMENT:
water rinses and oil massages

Dislikes

CUT:
unimaginative, trendy cuts

COLOR:
highlights designed to look "natural"
hiding gray

STYLE:
perms
conformity
monotony

TREATMENT:
shampooing

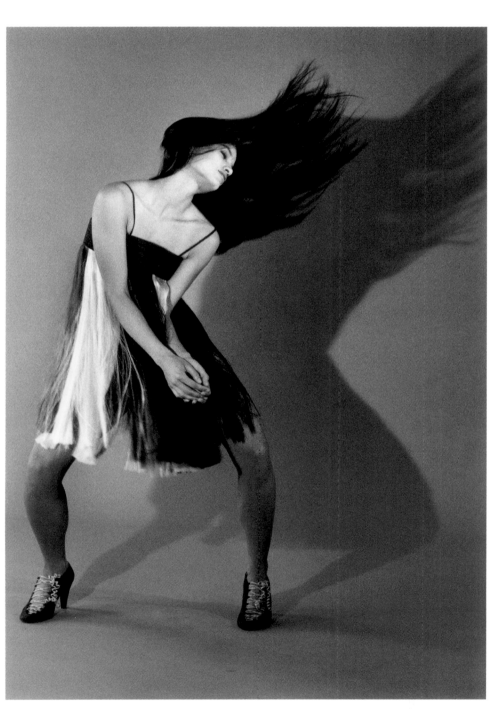

Giani, photographed by José Arman Pita for *Interview*. Courtesy *Interview*

"Ingrid Sischy, Interview's editor-in-chief, asked me to do a hair story and I thought I'd do hair clothes instead of hairdos."

Nadja Auermann, photographed by Mario Testino for *Glamour*. Courtesy *Glamour*

"Real braids, but fake tatoos."

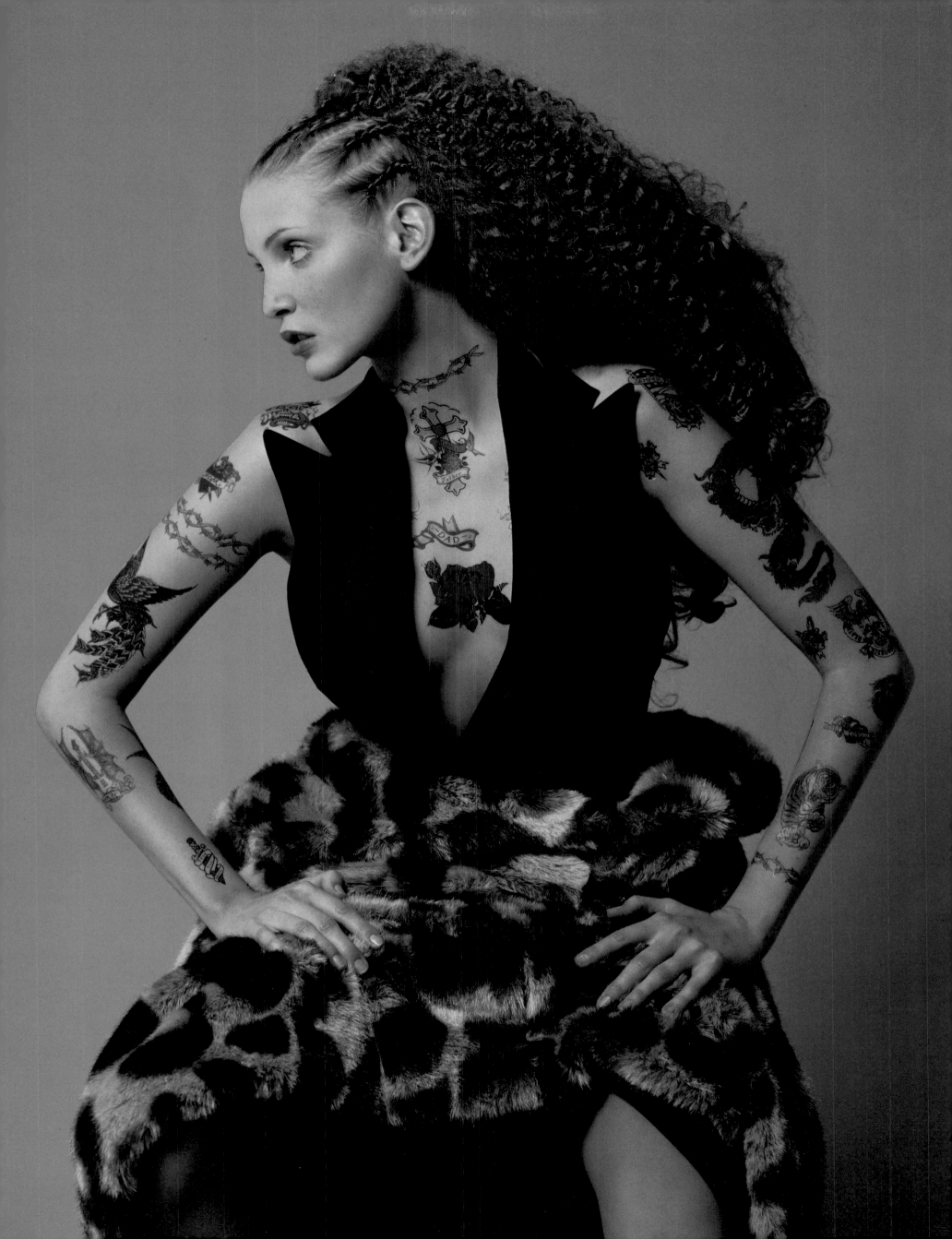

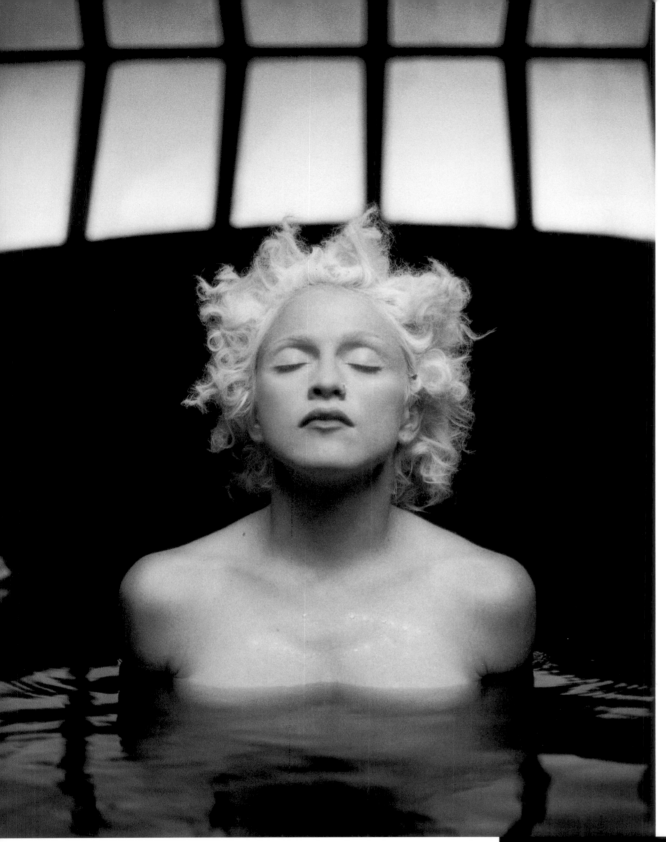

Clients

Madonna
Naomi Campbell
Bridget Hall
Nadja Auermann
Shalom Harlow

Madonna, photographed by Mark Romanek for her music video, *Bedtime Stories*

"The inspiration for this look was cotton candy."

Do's & Don'ts

While there are different techniques for creating different looks; for example, a curling iron will curl hair and hair spray will hold a style; I do not believe that there are rules as to what looks good. That is determined by the individual, the style of the clothes, the photographer, or whatever. It's all about the end result.

In any case, I was not properly trained myself, so I don't always do things the conventional way. Sometimes, one can even use toilet rolls as curlers. Things that I was completely opposed to in the past, like tacky, synthetic wigs and electric rollers, I later found pleasing uses for.

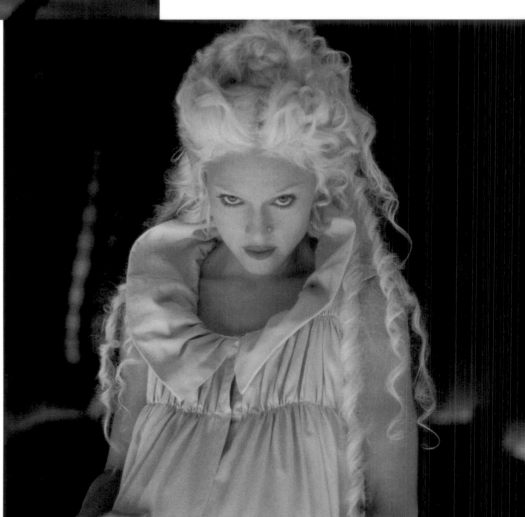

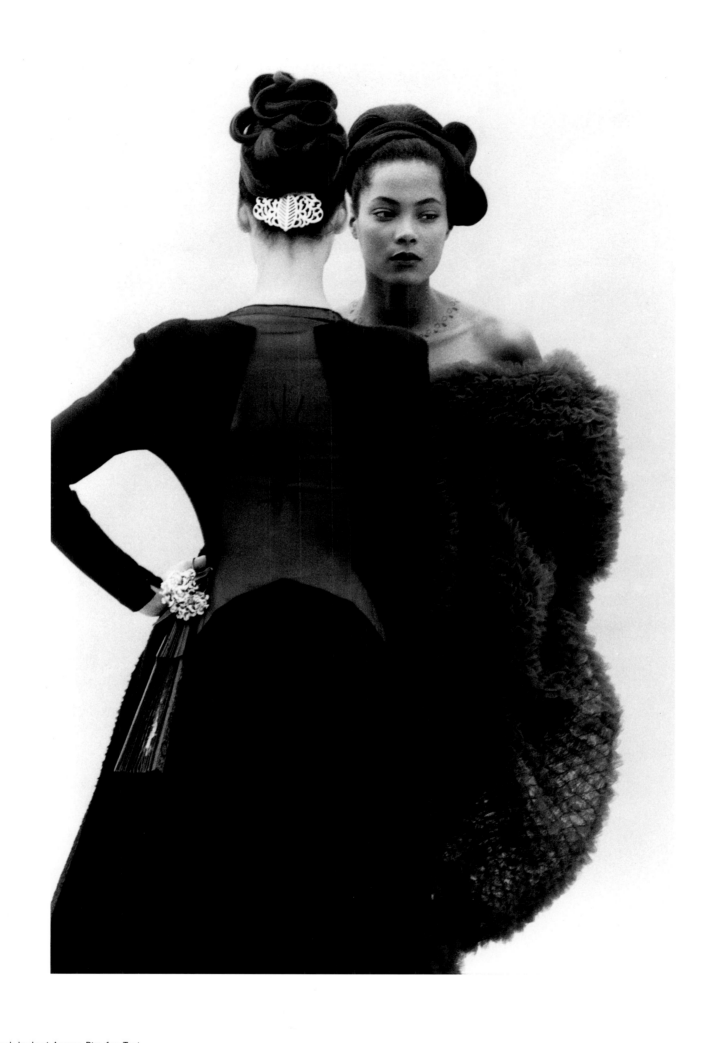

Photograph by José Arman Pita for *Taxi*

"I was inspired by soft-swirl ice cream."

JOHN SAHAG

Amazing Shapes

Serene and mysterious, the John Sahag Workshop floats two floors above the noise and chaos of midtown Manhattan. With its branching bamboo-shaped metal columns, organic stony stations, swirling terrazzo floors, and fishponds sunk into volcanic rock, the salon resembles either a fantasy design for a futuristic planet or a Paleozoic garden. Sahag himself, however – dressed for work in a black-ribbed T-shirt, black velvet pants, and black pointy-toed winklepicker shoes – appears completely of this day and age. He has the whippet-thin physique, shaggy hair, and intense, charismatic gaze of a rock star. But he also has the manners of a gentleman – honed, no doubt, by many years of soothing and serving a female clientele.

He is about to go to work on one of his loyal customers, a Venezuelan beauty with a full, unruly mane of blonde hair. Though it is already seven o'clock in the evening, Sahag takes no notice of the time. The other night, he says, he was "tapering Naomi Campbell's hair until three o'clock in the morning." He is infatuated with his *métier* and, in particular, obsessed with his technique, which he is about to demonstrate on his patron. Her hair has already been shampooed and dried straight. The whole Sahag method, which he invented 15 years ago, is predicated on the dry cut. "After all, you wear it dry," he says. "Hairdressers who cut wet retouch after they see it dry anyway." First, he discusses length with the woman. "It is so important to agree with the lady about length," he says. "After that's settled, the question is how to carve it." Sahag habitually speaks in the language of sculptors; "the idea, with hair or sculpture, is to make beautiful shapes." Next, he pins the client's hair up in sections, leaving only the layer closest to the neck hanging free. He straightens that curtain of hair with a curling iron ("always silver – I can't stand gold"), and begins to snip and notch the ends into a meticulously calibrated

Jenny Brunt, photographed by Michael Thompson for German *Vogue*. Courtesy German *Vogue*.

"I felt this beauty shot needed clean, sparkling texture, so I played with gels."

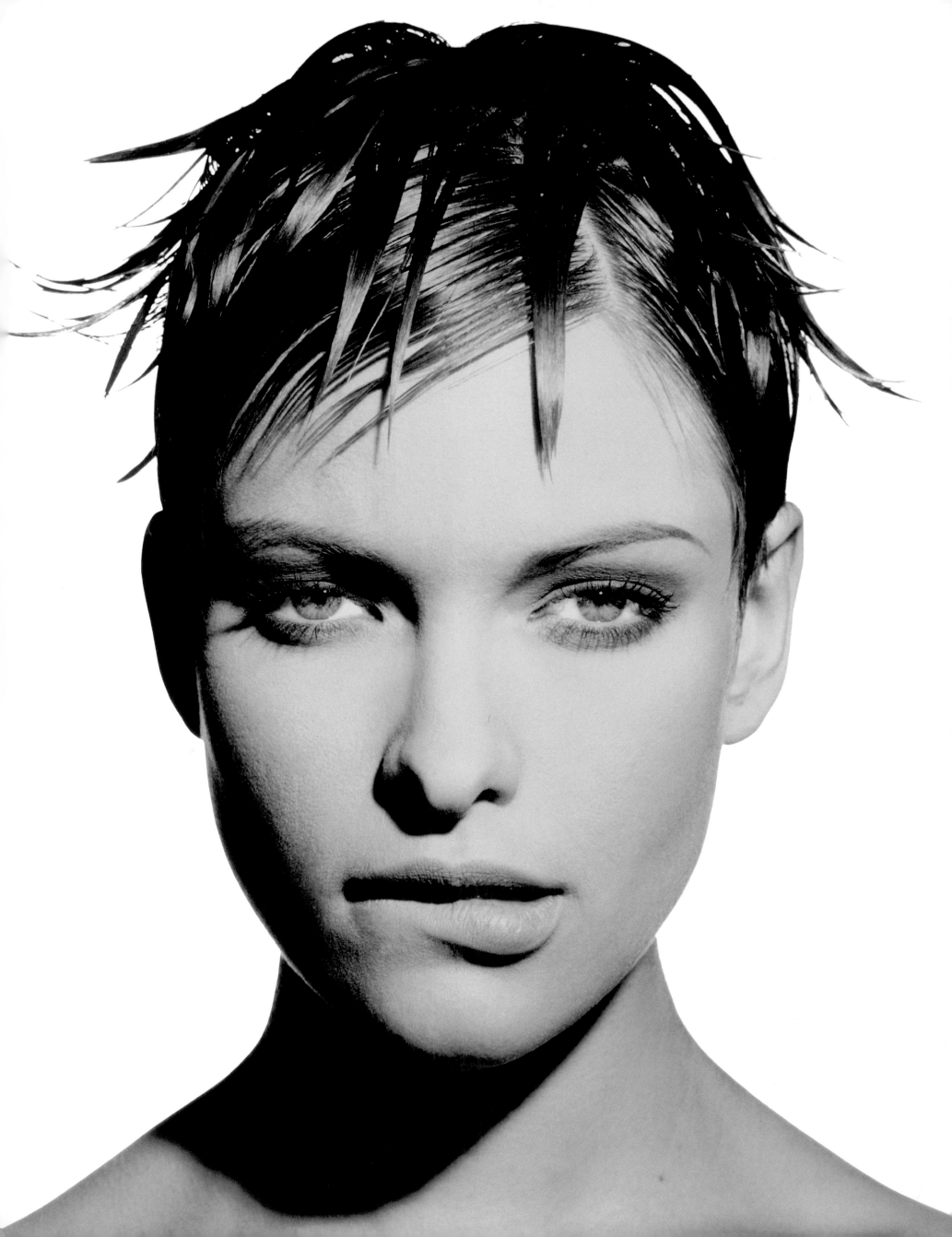

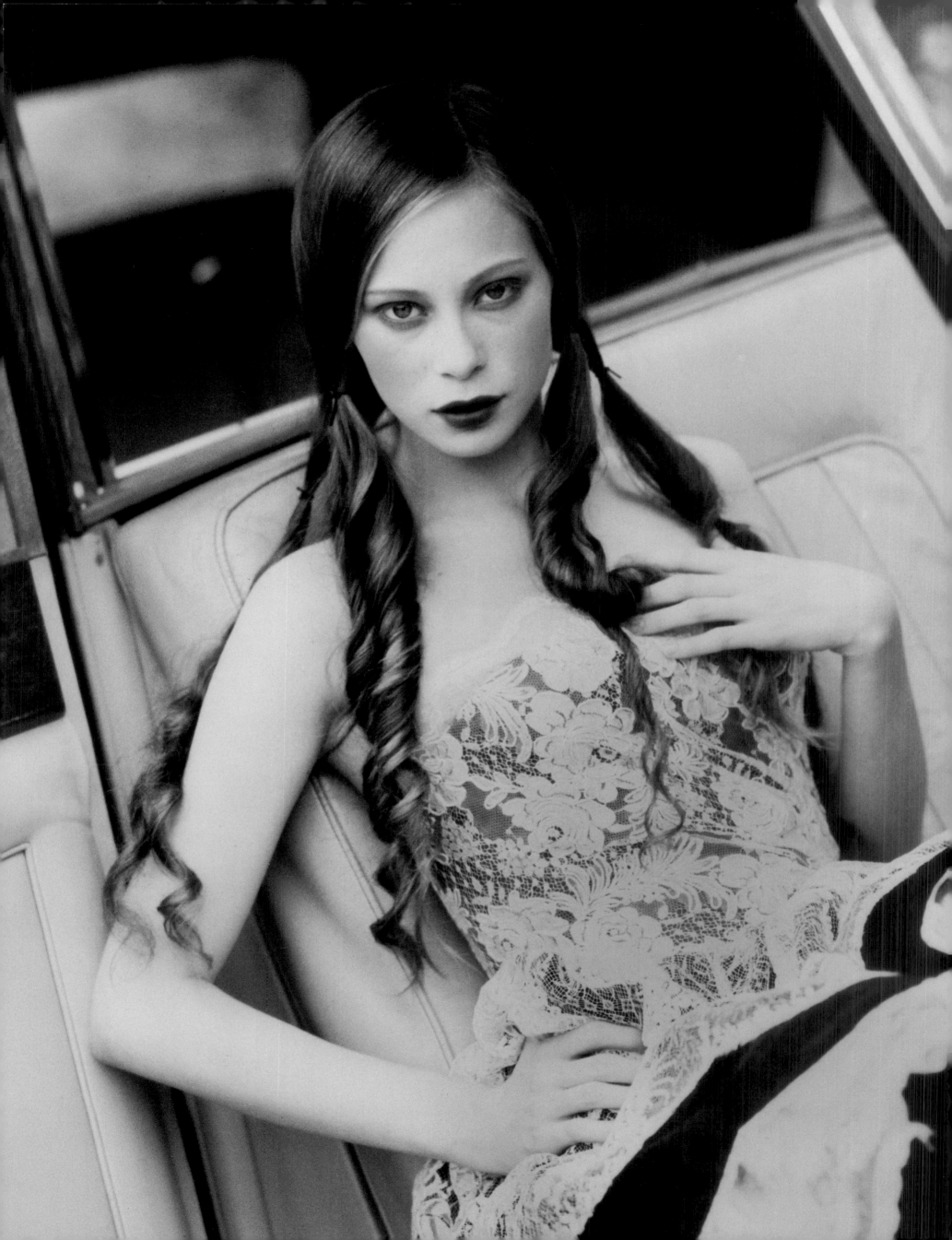

uneven line. "Cutting hair while it's straight is a more precise way of shaping it. You get to see every section, and know how it's going to fall. I keep ends soft as I'm taking the length off. I do not like the machine-made look of very blunt-cut hair. An irregular line is more beautiful than a straight one." Sahag proceeds section by section, layer by layer, varying each one slightly in length and in shape. "You get shifting weights through layering. Layering gives movement to hair." The hair becomes a series of transparent veils, swinging lightly and freely, one over the other. If each layer were the same length and shape, Sahag explains, the hair would become stagnant, leaden.

By the time Sahag has worked his way from the innermost to the topmost layer, and onto the bangs, almost an hour has elapsed. "You don't come here to rush," the client says. Adds Sahag, "It's not about time. It's about making amazing shapes. I do it as much for myself as for the lady. I carve every section for the end result, keeping 100% control. This way, the bangs, the tapering, the transparency – how much skin shows through hair – are all perfect." The client concurs. "I'm feeling much lighter now," she says, and, indeed, her golden hair seems to radiate from her face like materialized sunshine.

Sahag's expertise evolved over many years, and in almost as many places. "Destiny controlled me," he says. It also arranged for him to be born to Armenian parents living in Beirut. His father catered to sybaritic Lebanese tastes by working in *haute couture*, while a close family friend, whom Sahag calls "the Alexandre of Beirut," operated one of the city's poshest beauty parlors. Starting at age 8, Sahag worked during the summer holidays in this "super luxurious salon," sweeping floors "and breaking ashtrays." He was "flabbergasted" by the glamorous coiffures confected there. "The women were stunning. It was a period of great elegance." This idyll was interrupted, however, when Sahag's father, disturbed by political unrest in Lebanon, moved his family to Australia. "Dad said, 'We're going as far away as we can.' Australia seemed to him a new, young country, and my whole family is crazy about the sea. So he opened a couture shop in Sydney."

But, Sahag says, "the hair thing stayed in me so strong" that by age 14, he left school to attend a technical college and to work in a local salon. "My father also bought me a dryer and hired a friend to build a pastel blue Chinese lacquer station" – both of which he set up in his bedroom for "Sunday matinees." By 16, he was working for the Sydney branch of Alexandre, a position that inspired the Sydney *Morning Herald* to write him up as "the youngest senior hairdresser in the world." Searching for larger arenas, he moved first to Melbourne and then to Paris, promising his parents he would be back in six months. Desperate for a work permit, he lived rent-free in a garage, scavenging for work wherever he could find it. Yet, he says, "There was a fearlessness in me. I knew things would end up okay."

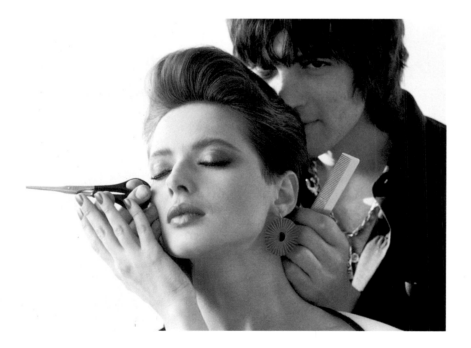

Hairstory

STYLIST: *John Sahag*
SALON ADDRESS: *The John Sahag Workshop, 425 Madison Avenue, New York City*
PLACE OF BIRTH: *Beirut, Lebanon*
FIRST JOB: *Age 8, sweeping floors at a hair salon*
TRADEMARK: *The dry cut with tapering*

John Sahag and Isabella Rossellini, photographed by Denis Piel for American *Vogue*. Courtesy American *Vogue* ©The Condé Nast Publications Inc.

Nina Brosh, photographed by Dominique Issermann for Italian *Vogue*. Courtesy Italian *Vogue*

"Here I used a curling iron."

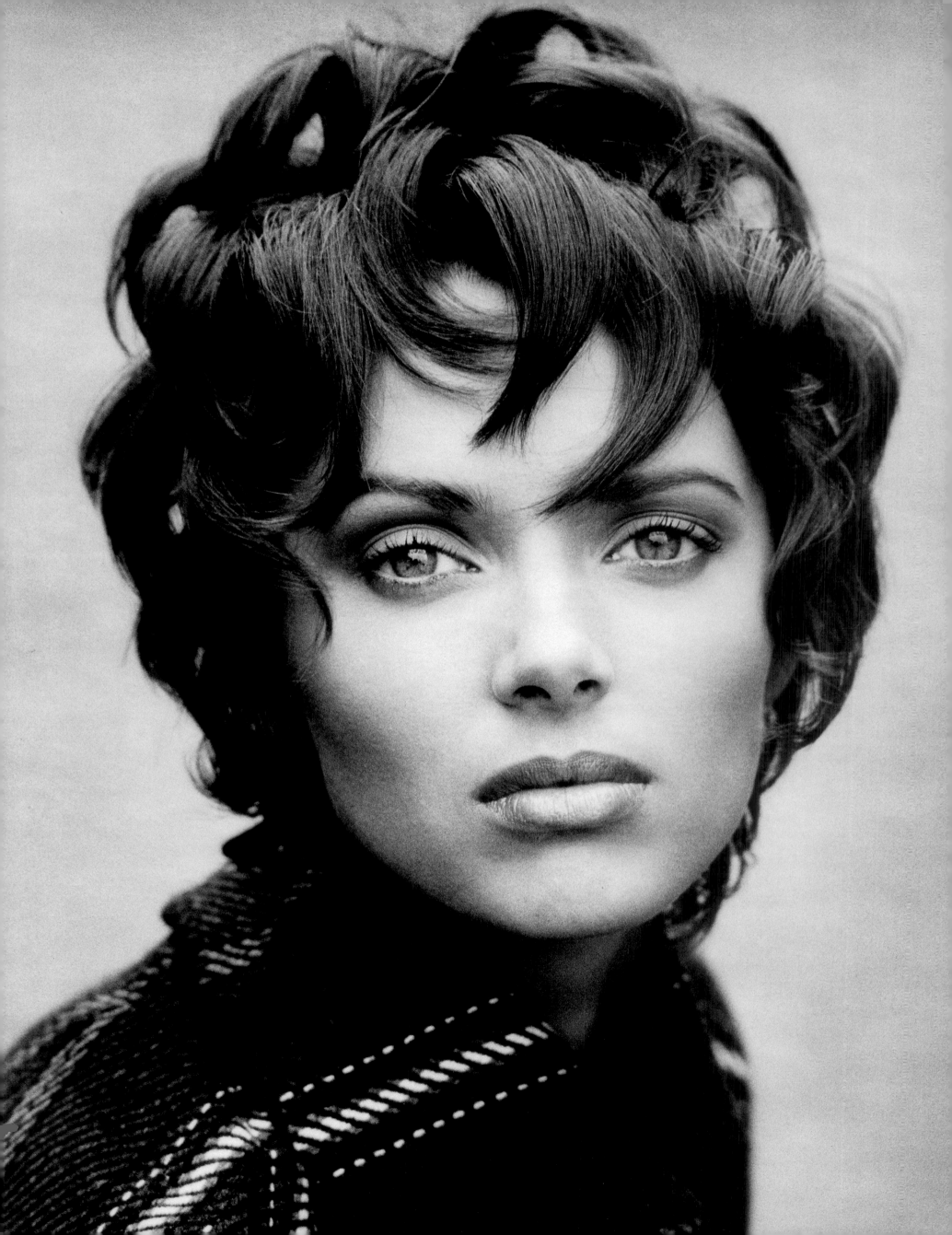

Through a combination of hard work, luck, and talent, he eventually landed a five-year contract as artistic director of the Maniatis Salon. Within months, he received his first editorial assignments with photographers Patrick Demarchelier, Gilles Bensimon, and Guy Bourdin for *Elie* and French *Vogue*. "Here I was, this young punk from the moon," he recalls, "suddenly doing well and thriving in the most glamorous part of the planet!" Helmut Newton spotted his work, and gave him his first cover, for *Stern* magazine. "I was just interested in doing amazing shapes, experimenting with how modern and edgy I could make them." Before long, magazines and advertisers had him shuttling regularly to Italy and then New York, where he finally settled in 1982. "For 14 years I had done only studio work. I must have been the first hairdresser to establish a career independent of any salon." But by 1985 he felt ready to open his own workshop, on East 53rd Street. In its atelier atmosphere, Sahag feels more at liberty to experiment and create – "I'm not directed by a fashion editor or ad agency" – and he relishes the opportunities to pass the Sahag technique on to his young assistants.

A nonprofessional can profit too from Sahag's instructive philosophy. For instance, Sahag sensibly advises that hair must always be cut into "a harmonious shape." He opposes anything that is "aging, contrived, or not modern" – such as a flip ("ridiculous") or a cotton-candy do. "I love things that you've never seen before. Like anything worthwhile, that's not so easy to achieve!" A good haircut, he believes, automatically "falls into a beautiful shape" after washing. If any styling is involved, Sahag teaches his client to master the method "with great speed." Most adamantly, he warns women to stay away from performing complicated chemical procedures, such as highlights or perms, at home. "I wouldn't do my own hair at home!" And he exhorts women not to be afraid to ask someone with wonderful hair where she goes for her cuts. "And if you feel the salon charges more than you can afford, consider that you'd spend at least as much on a dress that you take off at the end of the day." Trends toward long or short hair are, to him, completely irrelevant. The point is not the length, but "the shape and the carving." Finally, Sahag's "best advice" is to look after your hair with appropriate conditioners and treatments. "It's like taking care of teeth – preventive medicine is a necessity." Hair, he passionately feels, is "a mystical substance" that should be treated with reverence. "The amount I've learned about it, I should be 90 years old. But then again, there's still so much more to know!"

Facing page and right: **Heather Stuart-White,** photographed by Marc Hispard for *W.* Courtesy *W*

"Short, sexy hair never looks bad."

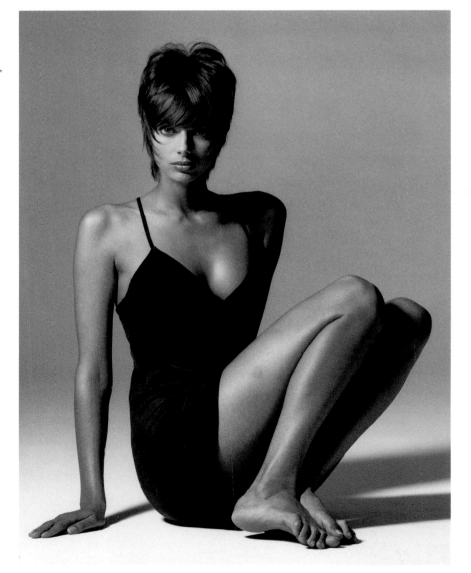

Do's & Don'ts

Avoid hairdressers who talk a lot, are constantly late, have a bad attitude, or make you feel that they are doing you a favor.

If your hairdresser is a sincere human being, love and trust him, or her, a little more.

Make sure your haircut looks modern and edgy, and suits your features, personality, and lifestyle.

Change your style at least twice a year.

Your hair color should be painted into a unique shade, which suits your skin tone, hair texture, and cut. It should also require only minimum maintenance.

Make sure you cleanse and condition your hair with the best possible products. It will be worth it.

It is a must to treat your hair with deep conditioners every four to six weeks.

Never wear contrived styles unless you are in show business, or have other theatrical reasons.

Ask your hairdresser about quick fixes (changes) of hairstyle.

For the right occasion, be daring with a more amazing style that fulfills your fantasies, and have it done by someone who shares your excitement.

Jenny Brunt, photographed by Michael Thompson for German *Vogue*. Courtesy German *Vogue*

"In haircutting, shapes are limited only by your imagination."

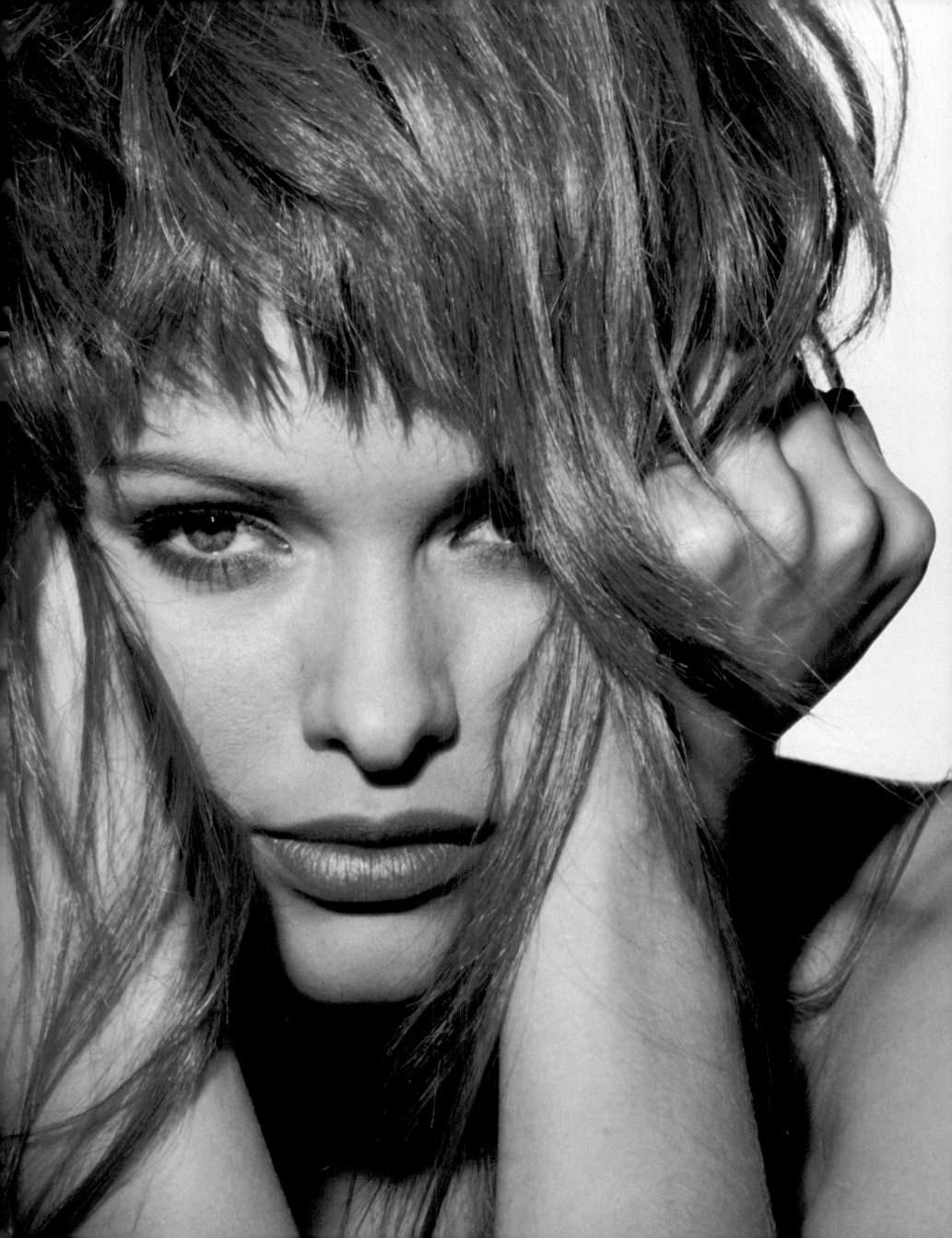

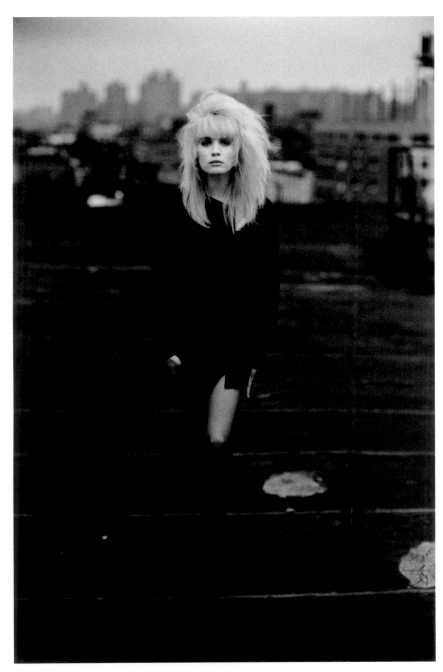

Lena Hyltof, photographed by Sante D'Orazio for Italian *Vogue*. Courtesy Italian *Vogue*

"Three different cuts in one long, dangerous look."

Likes

CUT:
finding a good stylist by asking strangers on the street who cut their hair
client and stylist to agree upon length before cutting begins
dry cuts
cuts with irregular lines and layers

COLOR:
using color (not bleach) for highlights and low-lights

STYLE:
stylist-client consultations about home styling

TREATMENT:
regular salon treatments
regular home conditioning

Dislikes

CUT:
any haircut that takes less than 40 minutes
blunt cuts
"flips"

COLOR:
bleached-in highlights
overbleached blondes

STYLE:
beehive coifs

Stephanie Seymour, photographed by Oberto Gili for *New York* magazine

"I shape and carve my own hairpieces."

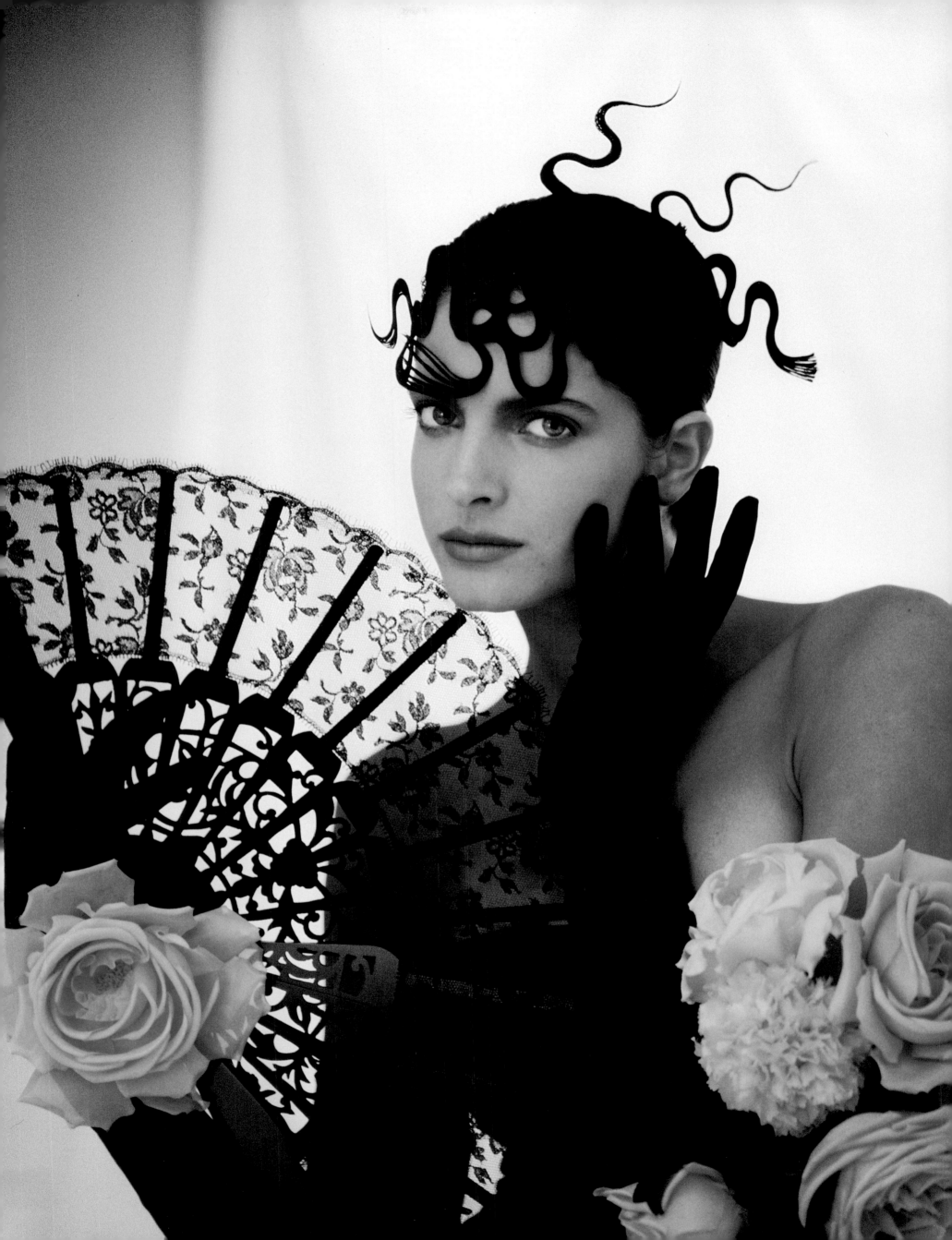

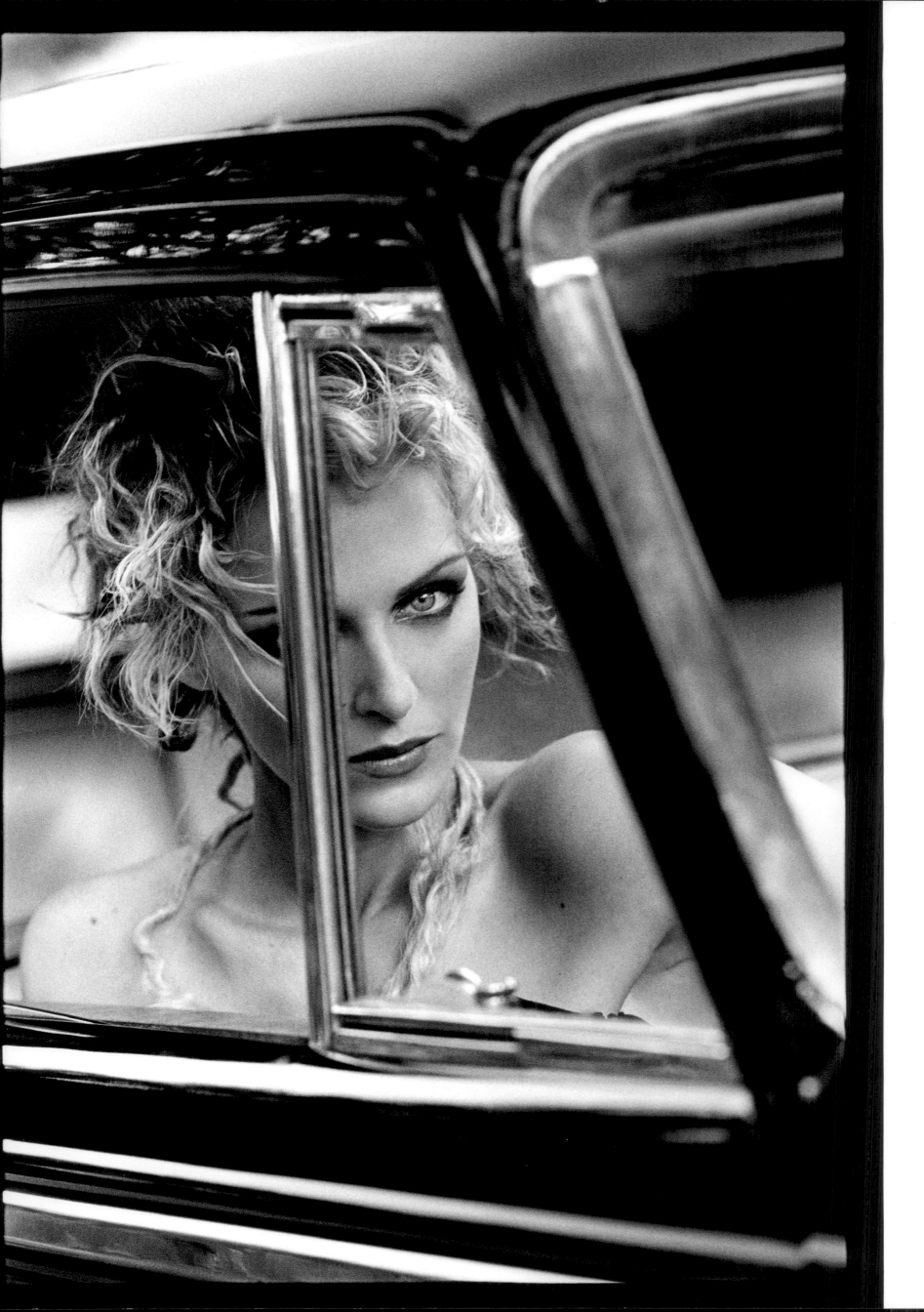

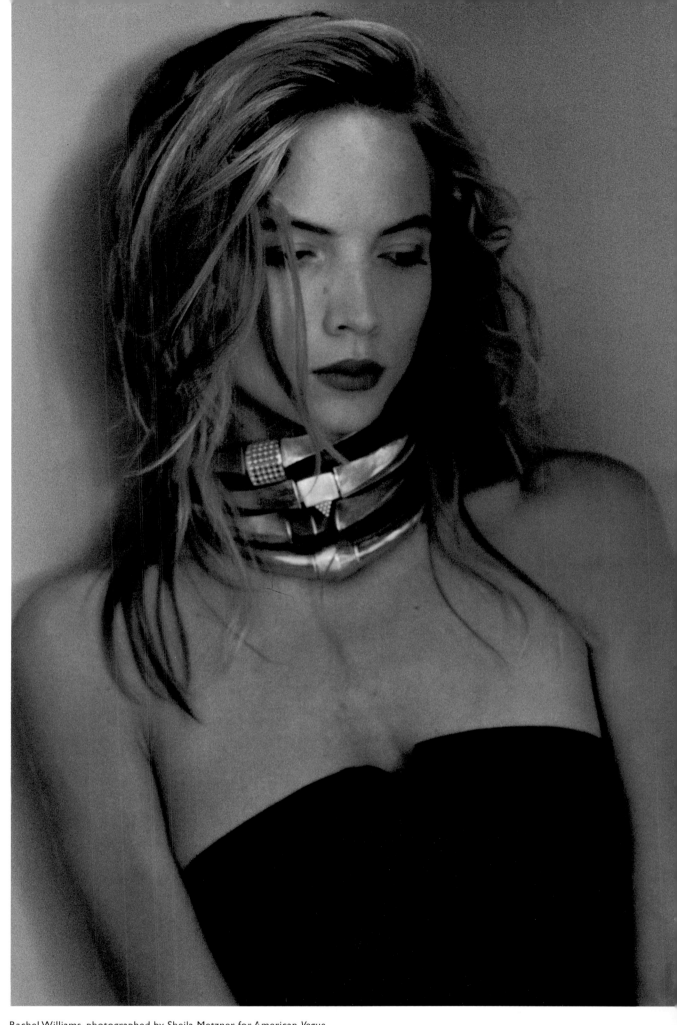

Rachel Williams, photographed by Sheila Metzner for American *Vogue*.
Courtesy American *Vogue* ©The Condé Nast Publications Inc.

"It's amazing what an iron can do."

Simonetta, photographed by Dominique Issermann for Italian *Vogue*. Courtesy Italian *Vogue*

"Drive-by style."

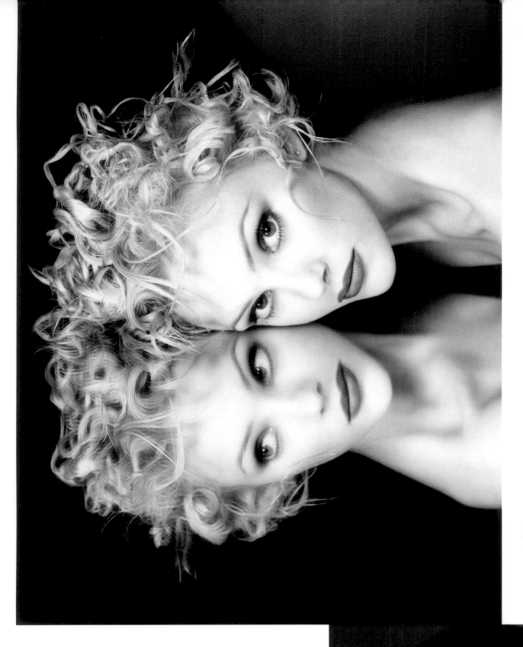

Clients

Julia Roberts

Bette Midler

Jack Nicholson

Farrah Fawcett

Bruce Springsteen

Raquel Welch

Demi Moore

David Lee Roth

Claudia Schiffer

Naomi Campbell

Brooke Shields

Isabella Rossellini

Jaime Richar, photographed by Albert Watson

"Subway folie."

Gina, photographed by Lorraine Sylvestre
for The John Sahag Workshop

"A multitextured, multicolored cut."

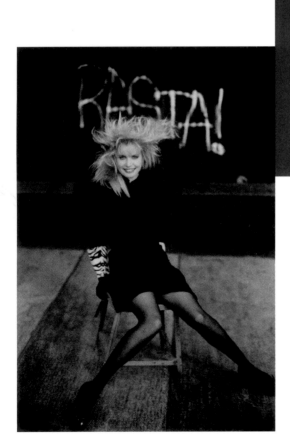

Lena Hyltof, photographed by Sante D'Orazio for Italian *Vogue*.
Courtesy Italian *Vogue*

"An abstract splash."

Yasmeen Ghauri, photographed by Albert Watson for German *Vogue*. Courtesy German *Vogue*

'The hair speaks for itself."

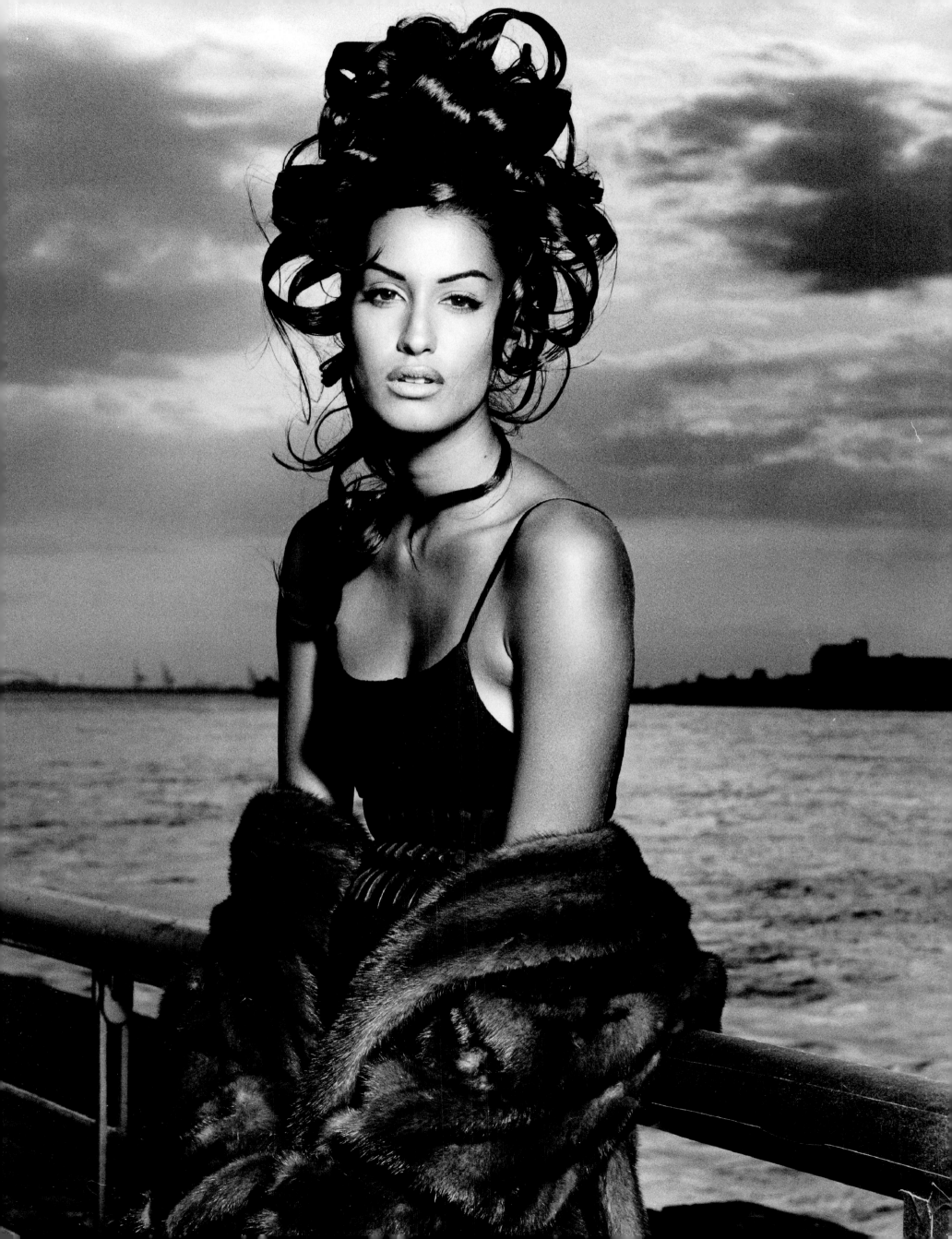

Shear Gratitude

AMY FINE COLLINS thanks:

First, Yves Durif for his wisdom and for finding the right hairstyle for me. Before Yves, I felt as if I was wearing someone else's hair on my head. I trust him so completely, I just sit in the chair and let him do with me as he pleases – a privilege I accord no other man!

Justine Rendal for telling me I had to do this book even if I had no time. Liz Tilberis for her participation. Joseph Montebello for his creative support. Paul Mahon and Aimee Bell, both for their sound advice. Marijke Smit and Maya Pettiford for their hard work. All the stylists and photographers whose generosity made this project possible. Annemarie Iverson and Deborah Curcio for their expertise. Caroline Flandrin and L'Oréal Technique Professionnelle for their foresight. Bradley Collins, Jr. for reading parts of the manuscript. Nicholas Callaway for his unparalleled vision.

Toshiya Masuda for his expert eye. Mary Trasko for her inexhaustable fund of knowledge. Ivan Wong, Jr. for his hair, which inspires us all. Christina Kulukundis for being the perfect editorial and research assistant to Antoinette White. Paula Litzky for her wealth of experience. True Sims for producing such a beautiful book. Monica Moran, Sophia Seidner, Andrea Danese, José and Nellie Rodríguez and Sang-Joon Kang for all their invaluable support.

Geoffrey Beene, Horst and Babs Simpson for endless inspiration. Miriam, Vivien, Gene and Robert for their abiding friendship.

Madonna for her behind-the-scenes help and enthusiasm.

And above all, the beautiful Antoinette White, an extraordinarily brilliant, courageous and graceful editor.

CALLAWAY EDITIONS thanks:

Photographers Patrik Andersson, Adel Awad, Mark Babushkin, Neal Barr, Gilles Bensimon, Juliette Butler, Eric Boman, Alex Chatelaine, Walter Chin, Lorraine Day, Sante D'Orazio, Patrick Demarchelier, Arthur Elgort, Hans Feurer, Oberto Gili, Marc Hispard, Dominique Issermann, Matthew Jordan-Smith, Karl Lagerfeld, Darryl Lane, Kevin Leong, Peter Lindbergh, Andrew Macpherson, Didier Malige, Raymond Meier, Steven Meisel, Sheila Metzner, John Peden, Irving Penn, Preston Phillips, Denis Piel, José Arman Pita, Yusuf Rashad, Mark Romanek, Paolo Roversi, Lord Snowdon, Melvin Sokolsky, Patrice Stable, Bert Stern, Wayne Summerlin, Lorraine Sylvestre, Jürgen Teller, Mario Testino, Michael Thompson, Ellen von Unwerth, Albert Watson, Bruce Weber, Timothy White, Eddie Wolfl and Firooz Zahedi.

Leslie Sweeney, Palma Driscoll, Allyn and Susan Magrino, Jean François Raffalli, Amy Kirkman, Timothy Priano, Jill Hunter and Helen Oppenheim.

L'Oréal Technique Professionnelle and Caroline Flandrin for their generous support.

Her Royal Highness, The Princess of Wales, Madonna, Ivor Frischknecht, Albert and Elizabeth Watson, George Andreou, Jun Kanai, Nicholas Mayer White, Gisela Mayer White, James Grodd, Victoria Wilson, Gordon Lish, Frank Maresca, Roger Ricco, Suki Buchman, Michael Gordon of Bumble and Bumble, Nick and Joseph of Bumble and Bumble, Kevyn Aucoin, Linda Wells, Diana Edkins, Tina Gaudoin, Sandy Arrowsmith, Marcey Engleman, Jed Root, Anthea Liontos, Nicolai Groessel, Walter Sassard, Matthew Cory Morgan, Richard Benson, Daniel Benson, Susan Winget and Tracy Feith, John D'Orazio, Igor Vishnyakov, Barbara Bergeron, Meredith Ward, Neal Durando, and Raoul Goff, Gordon Goff, Kelly Steis, Eric Ko and Ruby Sia of Palace Press International.

CHRISTIAAN thanks:

My father Jaap, the barber who made me touch and feel a head right. Yo Dad? Marianne, for longlive love. Arthur Elgort, freedom, independence, and Comedy Central. My teenboys Piet and Henk, "Yeah Dad." Polly Mellen, "Style, style, form, style." The girls who put their heads up.

JULIEN D'YS thanks:

Karl Lagerfeld, Peter Lindbergh, Juliette Butler, Patrick Demarchelier, Javier Valhonrath, Nick Knight, Michael Thompson, Kristen McMenamy, Kim Williams, Linda Evangelista, Jenny Haworth, Patricia Velasquez, Cecilia Chancellor, Marie Sophie Wilson, Naomi Campbell, Christy Turlington, Nadja Auermann, Uli, Lindsay, Cindy Crawford, Meghan Douglas, Nicoletta Santoro, Betty Bertramy, Elisabeth Dijan, Paul Cavaco, Florentine Pabst, Mako Yamasaki, Phebis Posnic, Camilla Nickerson, Stephane Marais, Linda Cantello, Kevyn Aucoin, François Nars, Heidi Morawetz, Comme des Garçons, Yohji Yamamoto, John Galliano, Chanel, Marion de Beaupre, Catherine Mathis, Tamaris, L'Agence Atlantis.

FREDERIC FEKKAI thanks:

My son, Alexander.

KHAMIT KINKS thanks:

Mr. Bronner who was fearless as a pioneer, his family, Janet Wallace and the staff at Bronner Brothers. Susan Taylor, Editor-in-Chief at *Essence,* for her vision. Mikki Garth-Taylor, cover and beauty editor at *Essence,* for making Khamit Kinks a well-known name not only in the hair industry but to black women all across the globe. We appreciate her good taste. Malaikia Hilton, the mother of exquisite braiding in America, who shared her knowledge and nurtured all those willing to learn. Nawili Ayo, who defined the fine art of hair beading, a bead master with a heart of gold. Dr. Eva Harden, the godmother of cosmetology who has fostered many under her wings. Sha Wafer, who taught us our first extension technique and who continues to support us and cheer us on. Maitefa Angaza, whose skillful writing talents were responsible for Khamit Kinks receiving national exposure in the early days. Last but definitely not least, to Vivian Baltrop and Barbara Baltrop Newsome, Annu's grandmother and mother, whose nurturing and hairdressing skills inspire her to this day.

DIDIER MALIGE thanks:

My mother, Josiane Malige, Grace Coddington, Liz and Andrew Tilberis, Bryan Bantry, Palma Driscoll, Jean Louis David, Angela de Bona, Hans and Dot Feurer, Jennifer Harris, Joe McKenna, Arthur Elgort, Margaret Gibbons, Wendell Myryama, Francesco Scavullo, Carol Shore, Bonnie Maller, François Nars, Lexington Labs, Mary Greenwell, Dick Page, Kevyn Aucoin, Bruce Weber, Paul Beck, Buffy Birrattella, Nan Bush, Callaway Editions, Mary Randolph Carter, Click Agency, Patrick and Mia, Paolo Roversi, Anna Harvey, Nancy Frederick, Donatella and Gianni Versace, Sheila Metzner and family, Lord Snowdon, Beatrix Miller, Steven Meisel, Patrick and Mia Demarchelier, all my friends at Ralph Lauren, Alain Pinon and Frederic Fekkai, my hairdresser.

SAM MCKNIGHT:

Very sincere thanks to all of you who have been involved since day one. You know who you are.

SERGE NORMANT thanks:

My parents and my sister Marina who have been so instrumental in my success thus far. The exquisite models, the makeup artists, and the photographers who portray my art. And, of course, my agent Timothy Priano who keeps my life sane.

ORLANDO PITA thanks:

Kevyn Aucoin, Paul Cavaco, Grace Coddington, Jo Anne Gair, Rory Gevis, Lori Goldstein, Marcelino Gonzalez, Tonne Goodman, Denise Markey, Polly Mellen, Laura Mercier, Heidi Morawetz, Moyra Mullholland, François Nars, Tom Pecheux, Jean François Raffalli, Ronnie Rivera, Karin Roitfeld, Paul Starr, Leslie Sweeney, Topolino, Ariella Vegliack, and above all my family.

JOHN SAHAG:

I would like to thank the fashion industry for inspiring me from a tender age, for giving me a chance and helping me grow by contributing to their dreams. All the fashion editors, fashion stylists, makeup artists and, of course, photographers must know that without you, my dreams could not have come true.

Colophon

Hair Style was produced by Callaway Editions, Inc.

Nicholas Callaway, Editorial Director and Publisher

Antoinette White, Editor

Toshiya Masuda, Designer

True Sims, Production Director

Paula Litzky, Associate Publisher

Monica Moran, Associate Publicist and Assistant to the Publisher

Sophia Seidner, Assistant to the Associate Publisher

Ivan Wong, Jr., José Rodríguez, and Sang-Joon Kang, Design and Production Associates

Christina Kulukundis, Editorial Assistant

Mary Trasko, Consultant

Barbara Bergeron, Neal Durando, Kelly Steis, and Meredith Ward, Copy Editors

The text and display typeface is Gill Sans. Gill Sans, a typeface inspired by Edward Johnston's type for the London Underground Railroad of 1916, was designed by Eric Gill in 1928. A humanist face meticulously patterned after classic roman character proportions, it quickly became the most popular sans-serif typeface in Great Britain.

This book was printed and bound by Palace Press International, Hong Kong, under the supervision of Toshiya Masuda and Raoul Goff.

Cindy Crawford, with hair styled by Maury Hopson, photographed by Eric Boman for German *Vogue*. Courtesy German *Vogue*

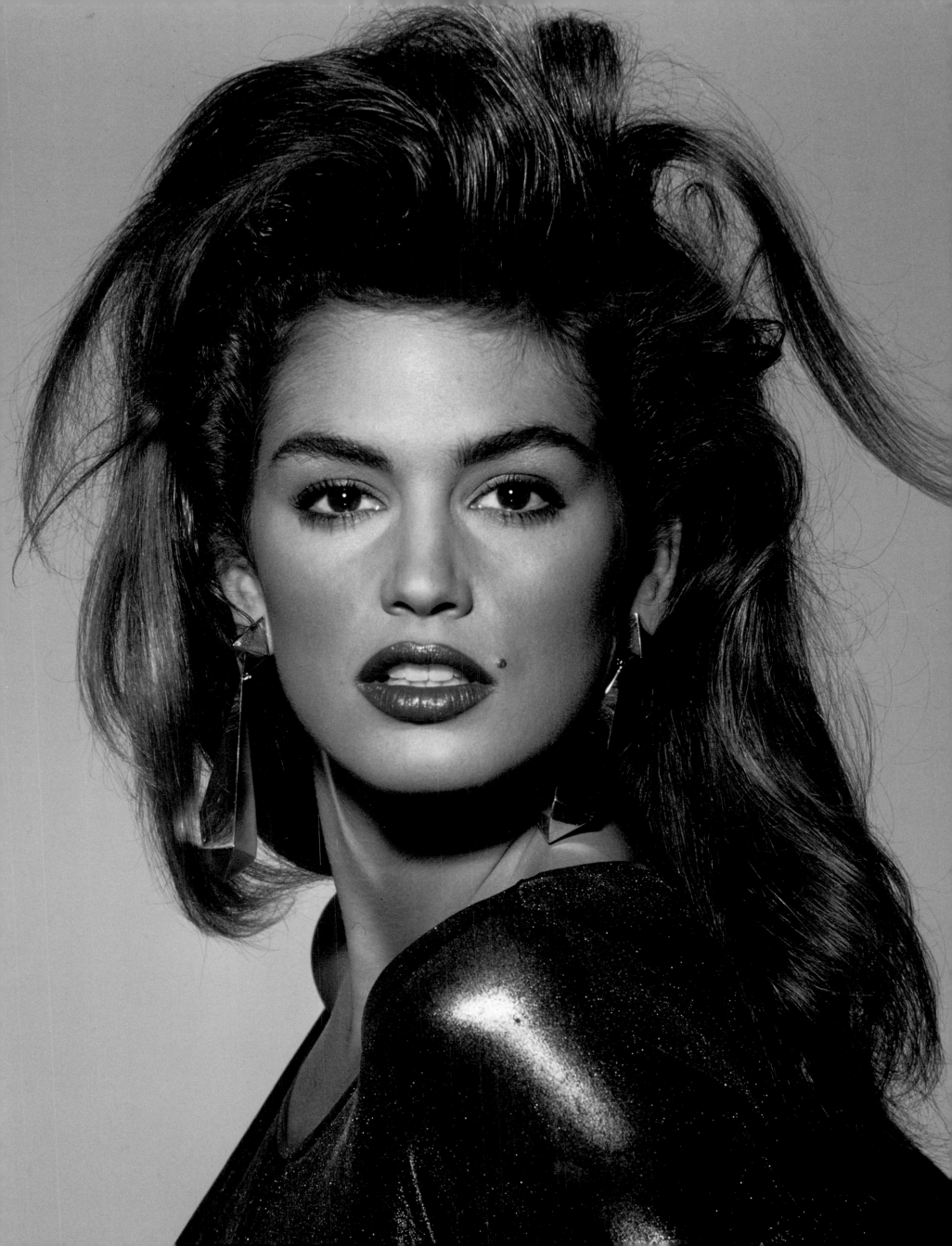